Clinical Governance

A Guide to Implementation for Healthcare Professionals

Rob McSherry

RGN, DipN (Lon), BSc (Hons), MSc, PGCE, RT

*Principal Lecturer, Practice Development
School of Health, University of Teesside
Middlesbrough*

and

Paddy Pearce

RGN, BSc (Hons), MSc

*Clinical Governance Manager
Northallerton Health Services NHS Trust
Northallerton, North Yorkshire*

with a contribution by

John Tingle

BA (Law Hons), MEd, Barrister

*Reader in Health Law
Director of the Centre for Health Law
Nottingham Trent, University
Nottingham*

Blackwell
Science

© 2002 by
Blackwell Science Ltd
Editorial Offices:
Osney Mead, Oxford OX2 0EL
25 John Street, London WC1N 2BS
23 Ainslie Place, Edinburgh EH3 6AJ
350 Main Street, Malden
MA 02148 5018, USA
54 University Street, Carlton
Victoria 3053, Australia
10, rue Casimir Delavigne
75006 Paris, France

Other Editorial Offices:

Blackwell Wissenschafts-Verlag GmbH
Kurfürstendamm 57
10707 Berlin, Germany

Blackwell Science KK
MG Kodenmacho Building
7–10 Kodenmacho Nihombashi
Chuo-ku, Tokyo 104, Japan

Iowa State University Press
A Blackwell Science Company
2121 S. State Avenue
Ames, Iowa 50014-8300, USA

The right of the Authors to be identified as
the Authors of this Work has been asserted
in accordance with the Copyright, Designs
and Patents Act 1988.

First published 2002

Set in 10/12.5 pt Sabon
by DP Photosetting, Aylesbury, Bucks
Printed and bound in Great Britain by
MPG Books Ltd, Bodmin, Cornwall

The Blackwell Science logo is a trade mark of
Blackwell Science Ltd, registered at the
United Kingdom Trade Marks Registry

For further information on
Blackwell Science, visit our website:
www.blackwell-science.com

DISTRIBUTORS

Marston Book Services Ltd
PO Box 269
Abingdon
Oxon OX14 4YN
(*Orders:* Tel: 01235 465500
Fax: 01235 465555)

USA
Blackwell Science, Inc.
Commerce Place
350 Main Street
Malden, MA 02148 5018
(*Orders:* Tel: 800 759 6102
781 388 8250
Fax: 781 388 8255)

Canada
Login Brothers Book Company
324 Saulteaux Crescent
Winnipeg, Manitoba R3J 3T2
(*Orders:* Tel: 204 837-2987
Fax: 204 837-3116)

Australia
Blackwell Science Pty Ltd
54 University Street
Carlton, Victoria 3053
(*Orders:* Tel: 03 9347 0300
Fax: 03 9347 5001)

A catalogue record for this title is available
from the British Library

ISBN 0-632-05801-3

Library of Congress
Cataloging-in-Publication Data
McSherry, Robert.
    Clinical governance: a guide to
implementation for healthcare
professionals/Rob McSherry and
Paddy Pearce; with a contribution by
John Tingle.
        p. ; cm.
    Includes bibliographical references and
index.
        ISBN 0-632-05801-3
    1. Medical care—Quality control.
2. Medical audit.   3. Clinical
competence.   I. Pearce, Paddy.
II. Tingle, John.   III. Title.
    [DNLM: 1. Quality Assurance, Health
Care.   2. Clinical Medicine—standards.
3. Medical Audit.   4. Patient Care
Management—standards.
W 84.1 M478c 2001]
RA399.A1 M375 2001
362.1′068′5—dc21

                                2001037951

Contents

Foreword

At the time of writing this Foreword, 'safety and quality' is the 'number one concern for the NHS as an organisation, and for everyone associated with it'. So announced Lord Hunt, Parliamentary Under Secretary of State for Health, at a Health Quality Service conference held at the Kings Fund in London on 19 July 2001.

Safety and quality go hand in hand. Safety is commonly regarded as the 'absence of unacceptable risk'. An organisation that pursues quality embeds sound risk management principles and processes into its systems and culture. Effective everyday management of unacceptable risk is an essential prerequisite for delivering quality.

But what exactly is quality? And what is the NHS agenda? Definitions of quality abound. Perhaps the simplest is 'conformance with requirements'. If the requirements for any health care product or service can be specified, and subsequently delivered, consistently, time after time, then you have a quality product or service. Thus the NHS quality fundamentally encompasses:

- clear national standards, such as those set out in National Service Frameworks (NSFs), NICE standards, controls assurance standards, and so on; and
- effective local delivery, co-ordinated through clinical governance, supported by the NHS Modernisation Agency, which incorporates the NHS Clinical Governance Support Team.

In addition, and 'closing the loop', the quality agenda is supported by:

- strong monitoring mechanisms, through the Commission for Health Improvement, the Performance Assessment Framework, the National Patient Safety Agency, and the Controls Assurance project; and
- measures for increasing patient and public involvement throughout the agenda.

Clinical governance brings the whole quality agenda together at a local level. Successfully implemented, clinical governance ensures that all the efforts of an organisation, and those that work in it, are focused and co-ordinated to deliver high and continuously improving standards of care and service. It is about changing the way people work, demonstrating that team working, leadership and communication, effective risk management, clinical effectiveness and active engagement with patients are all crucial to delivering better care.

This book skilfully pulls all of the essential components of clinical governance together, including a very useful chapter on legal considerations, and sets clinical governance within the wider corporate governance and controls assurance agendas. In the conclusion to Chapter 2 the authors argue that clinical governance is 'dependent upon successful integration of corporate governance and controls assurance' and that 'The challenge for the NHS is in "converging" all of the governance components under a single umbrella which all healthcare professionals can access, understand, implement and evaluate at a level most suited to their roles and responsibilities in the attempt to minimise risks'.

Current Department of Health policy is very much aimed at 'converging' or 'integrating' governance components. Indeed, Lord Hunt, in his speech at the Kings Fund on 19 July 2001, stated that:

> 'Clinical governance will be successful when we can drop the word "clinical", when everything a Trust does – not just the work of clinicians but everything from the portering to the catering, from the information provision to the human resources policies – are focused on delivering better, safer services to the patient.'

Perhaps 'healthcare governance', suggested in this book, is the umbrella term of the future?

But whatever the future for governance in the NHS, one thing is becoming increasingly clear. Quality of care in health care depends as much on the quality of systems and management as it does on the quality of individual clinicians. The emerging evidence from the growing patient safety field is that where patients are harmed during clinical care, the root causes of 'medical error' relate to systems and processes, and not poorly performing clinicians. Systems and processes are 'management' issues. The downside of not managing healthcare in the NHS in England is, among other things, one in twenty patients in secondary care suffering preventable harm leading to up to 40 000 unnecessary deaths and pro-longed hospital stay and additional treatment costs in excess of £2 billion per year. We need to *manage* healthcare better.

This is an excellent book. It sets out, clearly, the history and development of clinical governance and, from the authors' perspectives, based on

practical experience and a review of key literature, provides comprehensive practical guidance on implementation of clinical governance. It is an
essential text for all health care professionals. It breaks new ground in the
very important 'convergence' debate. As we grapple with modernising the
NHS, creating cultural change, shifting the balance of power, replacing
bureaucracy with accountability, improving the safety and quality of care
for patients, and improving conditions and prospects for NHS staff, I hope
that in the not too distant future we might see a follow-on publication that
truly integrates all the components of governance under the term
'healthcare governance'.

Stuart Emslie
Head of Controls Assurance
Department of Health

Preface

In our daily work as Principal Lecturer, Practice Development/Clinical Governance Manager, we are constantly being asked by staff for advice on what 'clinical governance' is and how to incorporate it into daily practice. Hence this introductory text, *Clinical Governance: A Guide to Implementation for Healthcare Professionals*, which addresses healthcare professionals' concerns about clinical governance, by providing a practical and simple guide based upon answering the following questions:

- Why is there a need for clinical governance?
- What is clinical governance?
- What are the key components of clinical governance?
- What are the legal implications of clinical governance?
- What are the barriers to implementing clinical governance in clinical practice?

We aim to answer the above by using reflective questions, activities and case studies taken from clinical practices to set clinical governance in context within today's health service. The information contained in the book is based upon a combination of the authors' clinical experiences, knowledge and understanding of 'clinical governance' derived from reading and reviewing the associated literature.

Rob McSherry
Paddy Pearce

Dedication

To my late parents Wilfred and Dorothy McSherry who I miss dearly. You are always in my thoughts and would have been proud to share this with me.

Rob McSherry

Chapter 1

Introduction and Background: Clinical Governance and the National Health Service

Rob McSherry and Paddy Pearce

Introduction

This chapter briefly describes the term 'clinical governance' and offers some possible reasons for its introduction into the National Health Service. The term 'clinical governance' became prominent following the publication of New Labour's first white paper on health, *The New NHS Modern, Dependable* (DoH 1997). Within this document the government sets out its agenda of modernising the National Health Service (NHS) by focusing on quality improvements. Clinical quality is rightfully assigned centre stage by 'placing duties and expectation on local health-care organisations as well as individuals' (DoH 1997, p. 34) to provide clinical excellence. The vehicle for delivering clinical quality is termed 'clinical governance' which 'is being put in place in order to tackle the wide differences in quality of care throughout the country, as well as helping to address public concern about well-published cases of poor professional performance' (Kings Fund 1999, p. 1). No single factor can be isolated that led to the development of clinical governance within healthcare, except that it attempts to revive a failing NHS and accommodate many societal and cultural changes, as highlighted in Activity box/Feedback 1.1.

Background

Why the need for clinical governance?

The literature offered by Scally and Donaldson (1998), Harvey (1998) and Swage (1998) seems to attribute the need for clinical governance to a decline in the standards and quality of healthcare provision, a point reinforced by the government. 'A series of well publicised lapses in quality have prompted doubts in the minds of patients about the overall standard of care they may receive' (DoH 1997, p. 5). Upon reviewing the literature on clinical governance we have noted that a key question has not been fully addressed in establishing why there is a perception of decline in standards and quality. The reasons for this perception could be that healthcare professionals and the public are more informed, better educated and more interested in health related issues and want a high quality service provision. Alternatively, quality and clinical standards have taken a back seat to other financial and resource management issues. Within this chapter it is our intention to explore the factors that may have contributed to the introduction of clinical governance.

Activity 1.1: Reflective question

Write down the factors that you feel may have led to the introduction of clinical governance.

Read on and then compare your findings with those in the Summary section at the end of the chapter.

It would be fair to say that there is no single factor that has led to the government's current position for modernisation. We could argue that patients' and carers' expectations and demands of all healthcare professionals have significantly increased over the past decade. This may be a result of increased public awareness of healthcare provision, facilitated by the publication of significant documents, notably *The Patient's Charter* (DoH 1992) and *The Citizen's Charter* (DoH 1993), both of which are freely available to the public. The charters may have, on the one hand, increased patients' and carers' expectations of healthcare, by offering information about certain rights to care. On the other hand the responsibilities of the patients to use these rights in a responsible way have been over used, resulting in higher demands for care and services in an already busy organisation.

In addition, other contributing factors such as changes in health policy, demographic changes, increased patient dependency, changes in healthcare delivery systems, trends towards greater access to healthcare information, advances in health technology, increased media coverage of healthcare and rising numbers of complaints going to litigation may have influenced the need for a unified approach to providing and assuring clinical quality via clinical governance (McNeil 1998).

Changes in health policy

In brief the NHS was established in 1948 following the passing of the National Health Services Act 1946 which committed the government at the time to fund the health service 'which rested on the principles of collectivism, comprehensiveness, equality and universality' (Allsop 1986, p. 12). The politicians at the time thought that addressing the healthcare needs of the public would subsequently reduce the amount of money required to maintain the NHS, the assumption being that disease could be controlled. However this was not the case. The NHS activity spiralled resulting in uncontrollable year-on-year expenditures to meet the rise in public demand for healthcare. In an attempt to manage this trend, the government introduced the principles of general management into the NHS via the Griffiths Report (Griffiths 1983). The philosophy of general management was concerned with developing efficiency and effectiveness of services. The rationale behind this report was to provide services that addressed healthcare needs (effectiveness) within optimal resource allocation (efficiency).

The report:

> 'recommended that general managers should be appointed at all levels in the NHS to provide leadership, introduce a continual search for change and cost improvement, motivate staff and develop a more dynamic management approach.'

> (Ham 1986, p. 33)

Key organisational processes were identified as missing in the report:

> 'Absence of this general management support means that there is no driving force seeking and accepting direct and personal responsibility for developing management plans, securing their implementation and monitoring actual achievement. It means that the process of devolution of responsibility, including discharging responsibility to units, is far too slow'

> (Griffiths Report 1983, p. 12).

This approach, whilst noble at the time, was concerned with organisational, managerial and financial aspects of the NHS, to the detriment of other important issues such as clinical quality. This style of management further evolved with the introduction of the white paper *Working for Patients* (DoH 1989), culminating in the development of a 'market forces' approach to the organisation and delivery of the healthcare services by the creation of a purchaser and provider spilt.

Health authorities and general practitioner fund holders were allocated resources (finances) to purchase care for their local population at the best price. It appears that the purchaser/provider split discouraged collaborative working and partnerships in the endeavour to develop quality services because the emphasis was directed towards financial performance. These imbalances led to the introduction of the white papers *The New NHS Modern, Dependable* (DoH 1997) and *Quality in the NHS* (DoH 1998a), putting clinical quality on a par with organisational, managerial and financial aspects of healthcare via 'clinical governance' – a framework 'which is viewed positively by many healthcare professionals as an ambitious shift of focus by the current government in moving away from finance to quality' (McSherry & Haddock 1999, p. 114). This approach to providing healthcare services places a statutory duty to match moral responsibilities and harmonises managers' and clinicians' responsibilities/duties more closely in assuring clinical and non-clinical quality. The impact of these reforms (DoH 1989, 1997, 1998a) has been to enhance public awareness and expectations for the NHS, placing an emphasis on achieving clinical quality.

Raising patient/carer expectations

The Patient's Charter (DoH 1992) *Raising the Standards* was distributed to all householders in the United Kingdom (UK) detailing the patients' and carers' rights of healthcare. The main principles behind this charter were that of informing and empowering the patients. This charter led to patients being viewed as consumers of healthcare. As consumers they are entitled to certain rights and standards of care. These standards included the right to be registered with a general practitioner, and as an inpatient to have a named consultant and qualified nurse, and the right to be seen within thirty minutes of any specified appointment time with a healthcare practitioner.

The Patient's Charter reinforced the aims of the Citizen's Charter (DoH 1993) by empowering the individual to become actively involved in the delivery of health services by the granting of certain rights. This style of healthcare delivery was unique, as previously patients tended to be seen as passive recipients of often-paternalistic methods (the 'doctor knows best') of providing care.

The benefit of these charters has been variable. Some individuals (public and healthcare professionals) are unaware of their existence in promoting raised standards, while many patients/carers are much more aware and informed of certain rights to treatments and healthcare interventions. In general, the majority of healthcare professionals have taken up and accepted the challenges posed by these charters in improving the delivery and organisation of healthcare. This can be evidenced by reviewing outpatient waiting time results, hospital league tables and the introduction of the named qualified nurse within inpatient settings. It could be argued that the Patient's Charter has led to a more questioning public about their rights and expectations of healthcare, such as: What is the problem? How will the condition be treated? What are the alternatives? What are the potential risks and benefits of all treatment options? These are genuine concerns for the public that need addressing.

The weakness of the Patient's Charter was raising rights and expectations to healthcare services which at times are difficult to achieve for many healthcare trusts. For example, to have a named qualified nurse assess, plan, implement and evaluate care from admission to discharge was impractical and overestimated. Similarly it is difficult for all outpatient attendees to be seen by their consultant on every visit. The consequence of raising expectations which are not achievable is dissatisfaction with services and higher incidence of complaints. The principles behind the charters are plausible providing the services are resourced sufficiently. Furthermore the publication of the Patient's Charter waiting times and league tables has highlighted inequalities in the provision of healthcare by demonstrating good and poor performers of services. For example, access to services for day case surgery could be variable according to region or demographic status of the local population and geography.

League tables alone do not provide the public with the background information of the local community health trends or the availability of healthcare services for individual Trusts, hence the disparity of service provision between Trusts. It may be inappropriate to perform day case surgery for hernia repairs in a hospital situated in a rural area with a large elderly population because of accessibility of services and appropriateness of the surgery to the patients' needs. This is more evident in society today with an ever increasing elderly population with multicomplex physical, social and psychological needs placing yet further demands on the health service, making the Patient's Charter standards more difficult to achieve.

Increased patient dependency

The increasingly ageing population means that patients are being admitted to acute and community hospitals with far more multicomplex physical and social problems (McSherry 1999), requiring timely appropriate interventions from a wide range of health and social care practitioners. For example the average length of stay in an acute hospital following total hip replacement surgery has gone down from fourteen to seven days, attributed to multidisciplinary and cross-agency collaborative working. A further example is in the advances in stroke care and rehabilitation and in the establishment of specialist stroke units where the evidence (Warlow *et al.* 1998) clearly demonstrates that recovery is better if these patients are managed in a specialist unit and not on an acute general medical ward.

The major effect of rises in dependency levels has been the need for greater efficiency, for example in maximising lengths of stay and maintaining high levels of acute bed occupancy. However, the shorter average lengths of patient stay seem to suggest that effective discharge planning is lessened due to staff having less planning time (particularly in complex social cases). Re-admission rates may have increased and certainly higher and greater demands are made of the community nursing services, hospital at home schemes and continuing and long term care facilities, as more patients with complex physical and social needs require continued healthcare.

Demographic changes in society

Health of the Nation (DoH 1991) suggests that life expectancy will increase for all. If this is the case it is inevitable that the NHS will become pressurised to provide more acute and continuing care services for an even larger elderly population. In an attempt to reduce healthcare demands, *Health of the Nation* sets targets for reducing morbidity (disease and disability trends) by concentrating on health promotion and disease prevention; for example, the reduction of strokes by the active management of high blood pressure (hypertension) and the reduction of deaths attributed to coronary heart disease by promoting healthy eating and exercise and where necessary the prescription of 'statins' (cholesterol lowering drugs) (DoH 2000).

The general population changes indicate that there has and will continue to be a large increase in the numbers of people living to and beyond 65, 75 and 85. Longevity seems to be on the increase for all (DoH 1991), reinforcing the growing trends of high dependency patients.

Advances in health technology

Advances in healthcare technology have made inroads into improving the quality and standards of nursing care delivery; for example, pressure relieving equipment, moving and handling equipment, medical administration and monitoring equipment and wound care management. All have the potential for enhancing the quality of care delivered by healthcare professionals. However, credentialisation (demonstrating the evidence that staff have the knowledge, competence and skills to use the equipment safely) may be questionable. The downside is allowing the staff time and resources for education and training to use the equipment in an ever demanding and stressful clinical environment. The latter should not be the case if clinical governance is implemented successfully. These identified pressures being placed upon healthcare professionals to deliver a high quality service based upon appropriate evidence, have the potential to create a conflict between balancing efficiency and effectiveness and maintaining quality and standards. These aspirations cannot be achieved for all patients and carers without adequate resourcing and government backing and some cultural changes.

Changes in care delivery systems

With the increases in the numbers of patients admitted with multiple needs, healthcare providers have had to change the pattern of care delivery in order to accommodate this growing need, leading to the development of acute medical and surgical assessment units, pre-operative assessment units, multiple needs and rehabilitation units, acute mental health assessment units, etc. This style of service provision seems to be about maximising the use of acute and community beds and encouraging collaborative working between primary and secondary care in the management and maintenance of the patient in the most appropriate setting; for example, in the shared care approach to the management of patients who have diabetes, where the care is shared between the GP and consultant endocrinologist with the backing of the diabetic team (diabetes nurse specialist, dietitian, podiatrist, ophthalmologist and pharmacist).

Initiatives such as hospital at home schemes (where possible maintaining the patient in their own home) are beginning to be developed along with public and private sector partnerships (acute illness managed in hospital with rehabilitation continued in a private nursing home until ready for discharge).

The driving force behind these innovations could be attributed to the reduction in junior doctors' hours (DoH 1998b) and the possible effects of the European working time directive (Working Time Regulations 1998), culminating in the development of nurse practitioners particularly in busy areas such as acute medical admissions and accident and emergency departments. This concept was reinforced in the early 2000s by the introduction of nurse consultants. These changes to healthcare delivery are directed towards enhancing the quality of care and raising public confidence.

Lack of public confidence because of recent media coverage of poor clinical practices

The media has played a major role in increasing patients' and carers' awareness of the NHS by the publication of clinical successes and failures in the organisation – notably the Allitt enquiry and Bristol case. The Allitt enquiry involved an investigation of a qualified enrolled nurse working in a paediatric unit who was convicted of murdering four children and injuring nine others. This was done supposedly while caring for patients (MacDonald 1996). The Bristol case relates to a consultant paediatric cardiac surgeon who was found to have a death rate for paediatric heart surgery significantly higher than the national average. This only became known as a result of whistle-blowing (The Lancet 1998).

The impact of these failings and others seems to have resulted in a growing lack of public confidence with the health service, with a rise in the numbers of complaints proceeding to litigation (Wilson & Tingle 1999).

Rising numbers of complaints going to litigation

Over the past decade we have witnessed a huge rise in the numbers of formal complaints made by patients and carers about hospital and community services which proceed to litigation. The estimated cost of clinical negligence for 2000–2001 is predicted to be around £500m (Wilson & Tingle 1999). These increased costs associated with litigation are attributed to:

- Increased activity levels of healthcare
- Greater propensity to pursue a complaint to litigation
- Increased compensations for negligence claims (more likely to seek redress when something goes wrong) if when patient sues the NHS they may be financially compensated.

It is worth noting here that the vast the majority of complaints are resolved at a local level, often with clarification, explanations and the occasional apology for when things have gone wrong. Honesty and openness are the key principles to deal with complaints, as well as the developing robust mechanisms for the sharing of information to deal with issues before they become problems (McSherry 1996). Management needs to encourage a learning culture which responds proactively rather than responding reactively to seek redress when something goes wrong. The ultimate aim is to have a blame-free culture that encourages healthcare professionals to openly report, discuss and learn from clinical incidents or clinical complaints. In many instances complaints arise from system failures rather than the actions or omissions of individuals. Healthcare professionals need to be made aware of this situation and have the knowledge, skills, competence and confidence to deal positively with complaints.

Trend towards greater access to healthcare information

The advances in information technology, for example the internet, have resulted in easier access to information by the public. Individuals are able to access the same information as healthcare professionals, for example, The Cochrane Library (http://hiru.mcmaster.ca/cochrane/cochrane/cdsr.htm; www.nelh.nhs.uk/cochrane.asp) and Department of Health website (http://www.doh.gov.uk/), empowering and informing the public with specific information relating to their condition. This ability to access information which was perhaps difficult to obtain previously is fuelling the public's demands and expectations for quality care.

Summary

Activity 1.1: Feedback

The contributing factors that have led to the introduction of clinical governance are some of the following:

- Changes in health policy
- Rising patient/carer expectations
- Increased patient dependency
- Demographic changes in society
- Advances in health technology
- Changes in care delivery systems

It is clear from Activity 1.1 that there are many contributing factors that have influenced the introduction of clinical governance within the NHS. Undoubtedly more factors will continue to arise, reinforcing the need for clinical governance in the future. It is therefore important that organisations and individuals embrace the concept of clinical governance in the pursuit of clinical excellence. This can only be achieved by having an understanding of where clinical governance originated and what it means in daily clinical practice, as outlined in Chapter 2.

KEY POINTS

- The reason for introducing clinical governance into the NHS was a perceived decline in clinical standards, service provision and delivery. This was reinforced by media coverage of major clinical failures

notably the Bristol Case and Allitt inquiry, resulting in a general lack of public confidence in their NHS.
- A more informed, consumer orientated public has greater expectations of the NHS, attributed to the different charters.
- Society is more questioning and litigious.
- A combination of societal, political, demographic and technological advancements have led to the introduction of clinical governance and the pursuit for quality in the NHS.

RECOMMENDED READING

Donaldson, L. J. & Muir Grey, J. A. (1998) Clinical Governance; A quality duty for health organizations. *Quality in Healthcare*, 7 (Suppl) S37–S44.

McNeil, J. (1998) Clinical governance: The whys, whats, and hows for theatre practitioners. *British Journal of Theatre Nursing*, 9(5) 208–16.

McSherry, R. & Haddock, J. (1999) Evidence based healthcare: Its place within clinical governance. *British Journal of Nursing*, 8(2) 113–17.

References

Allsop, J. (1986) *Health Policy & The National Health Service*. Longman, London.

DoH (1989) *White Paper: Working for Patients*. The Stationery Office, London.

DoH (1991) *Health of the Nation*. The Stationery Office, London.

DoH (1992) *The Patient's Charter; Raising the Standards*. The Stationery Office, London.

DoH (1993) *The Citizen's Charter*. The Stationery Office, London.

DoH (1997) *The New NHS Modern, Dependable*. The Stationery Office, London.

DoH (1998a) *Quality in the New NHS*. The Stationery Office, London.

DoH (1998b) *Reducing junior doctors' continuing action to meet new deal standards rest periods and working arrangements, improving catering and accommodation for juniors, other action points*. Health Services Circular 1998/240, Department of Health, London.

DoH (2000) *National Service Framework for Coronary Heart Disease: Modern Standards & Service Models*. Department of Health, London.

Griffiths, R. (1983) *NHS Management Enquiry*. Department of Health and Social Security, London

Ham, C. (1986) *Health Policy in Britain*. Macmillan, London.

Harvey, G. (1998) Improving patient care: Getting to grips with clinical governance. *RCN Magazine*, Autumn.

King's Fund (1999) *Briefing; What is clinical governance*. February. King's Fund, London.

The Lancet (1998) Editorial: First lessons from the 'Bristol case'. *The Lancet*, 351 (9117) 1669.

MacDonald, A. (1996) Responding to the results of the Beverly Allitt enquiry. *Nursing Times*, **92** (2) 23–5.

McNeil, J. (1998) Clinical governance: The whys, whats, and hows for theatre practitioners. *British Journal of Theatre Nursing*, **9** (5) 208–216.

McSherry, R. (1996) Multidisciplinary approach to patient communication. *Nursing Times*, **92**(8) 42–43.

McSherry, R. (1999) *Supporting patients and their families*. In *Caring for the Seriously Ill Patient* C. C. Bassett & L. Makin. Arnold, London.

McSherry, R. & Haddock, J. (1999) Evidence based health care: Its place within clinical covernance. *British Journal of Nursing*, **8** (2) 113–117.

Scally, G. & Donaldson, L.J. (1998) Clinical governance and the drive for quality improvement in the new NHS in England. *BMJ*, 317, 61–65.

Swage, T. (1998) Clinical care takes center stage. *Nursing Times*, **94** (14) 40–41.

Warlow, C., Van Gijn, J. & Sandercock, P. (eds) (1998) Stroke Unit Trialists' Collaboration. Organised inpatient (stroke unit) care after stroke. In *Stroke Module of the Cochrane Database of Systematic Reviews*. BMJ Publishing Group, London.

Wilson, J. & Tingle, J. (1999) *Clinical Risk Modification; a Route to Clinical Governance*. Butterworth Heinemann, Oxford.

Working Time Regulations (1998) The Stationery Office, London.

Chapter 2

What is Clinical Governance?

Rob McSherry and Paddy Pearce

Introduction

In Chapter 1 the contributing factors that led to the introduction of clinical governance were described and discussed. This chapter explores and explains where clinical governance originated, how this concept was introduced into the NHS and its implications for healthcare professionals, managers, Trust boards and organisations.

The evolution of clinical goverance

The term clinical governance can be traced to the white paper *The New NHS Modern, Dependable* (DoH 1997). This document outlines the New Labour government's strategy for the modernisation of the NHS, with clinical governance described as:

> 'a system which is able to demonstrate, in both primary and secondary care, that systems are in place guaranteeing clinical quality improvements at all levels of healthcare provision. Healthcare organisations will be accountable for the quality of the services they provide.'

> (McSherry & Haddock 1999, p. 113).

In essence, clinical governance in our opinion is viewed as the panacea for modernisation of the perceived failing NHS as reported in media coverage.

Prior to describing what the authors believe and understand to mean by the term clinical governance, a fundamental question requires answering. Where did clinical governance stem from?

Origins of clinical governance

Clinical governance evolved out of the term corporate governance, which originated primarily from the business world associated with the London

Stock Exchange. The intention of corporate governance in this instance was to safeguard shareholders' investments and companies' assets, the principle being that of protecting investors and minimising company risks from fraud and malpractice, e.g. the demise of Barings bank as a result of the practices of Nick Leeson (Chua-Eoan 1995). In an attempt to prevent similar incidents within the UK stock exchange, the Cadbury Committee was established. This committee reported in 1992 defining corporate governance as 'the system by which companies are directed and controlled' (NHS Executive 1999).

Cadbury identified three fundamental requirements to assure corporate governance within organisations:

- Internal financial controls, i.e. the annual auditing of financial accounts to ensure appropriate use of the company's finances without any underhand dealings.
- Efficient and effective operations, i.e. the company is providing value for money.
- Compliance with laws and regulations, i.e. health and safety is not being compromised; employers and public are protected.

This was termed the 'Cadbury Code'. This code was enhanced by the Greenbury and Hemple Committees, resulting in the publication by the London Stock Exchange of a *Combined Code of Principles of Good Governance*.

The code's major recommendations were that 'the board should maintain a sound system of internal control to safeguard shareholders' investments and company assets':

> 'The directors should, at least annually, conduct a review of the effectiveness of the group's systems of internal control and should report to the shareholders that they have done so. The review should cover all controls, including financial, operational, and compliance controls and risk management.'

> (NHS Executive 1999)

Basically this means that corporate governance is about having a systematic approach to demonstrate that the company is doing its best to protect the investors' monies and the company's future, and is complying with statutory obligations. To achieve this, all the company's operational processes require regular monitoring and reviewing in an open and transparent manner.

The Cadbury Code was improved by the Turnbull Committee, which reported in 1999 recommending the need for adequately resourced internal audit departments to evaluate risk and monitor the effectiveness of the company's performance. The potential benefits from corporate governance in the independent sector – open channels of communication, safeguarding public and employees, and demonstrating value for money – could equally be applied to the public sector. The government, in an attempt to demonstrate their commitment to improving public service provision, embraced the standards of corporate governance by introducing the principles of corporate governance into the NHS in 1994.

Corporate governance and the NHS

Activity 2.1

How do you think the principles of corporate governance may apply to the NHS?

Read on and then compare your responses with those in the Feedback box at the end of this section.

Corporate governance was introduced into the NHS via a three-stage process, which is continuing. This process is described here.

The development of a framework of corporate governance

This was outlined in the publication *Corporate Governance in the NHS; Code of Conduct and Code of Accountability* (NHS Executive 1999), where the focus of the document was directed at NHS Trust boards in ensuring and demonstrating that the conduct of the board was exemplary. The code of conduct for NHS boards is based on three principles shown in Box 2.1.

Box 2.1 Principles of corporate governance in the NHS

Accountability – everything done by those who work in the NHS must be able to stand the test of parliamentary scrutiny, public judgements on propriety and professional codes of conduct.
Probity – there should be an absolute standard of honesty in dealing with the assets of the NHS: integrity should be the hallmark of all personal conduct in decisions affecting patients, staff and suppliers, and in the use of information acquired in the course of NHS duties.
Openness – there should be sufficient transparency about NHS activities to promote confidence between the NHS authority or Trust and its staff, patients and the public.

DoH (1994)

Essentially the code of conduct and accountability is about ensuring that each member of staff knows who they are accountable to and for what practices. This should occur in an honest and open environment. Basically this means telling the truth when things go right and when things go wrong.

Improvements in the organisation and staffing of internal audit

This is about ensuring that internal systems are in place throughout the organisation that are working well in highlighting good practice and areas in need of improvement; for example, periodic auditing of staff expenses claims, and vetting the tendering process where external contractors are bidding for NHS work, to gain the best possible quote and ensure value for money.

The development of controls assurance

Controls assurance can be viewed as part of governance and is described as 'a holistic concept based on best governance practice' (NHS Executive 1999, p. 2); that means meeting the codes of conduct, and accountability as previously mentioned. Controls assurance is concerned with methods that enable healthcare organisations to provide evidence that they are doing their 'reasonable best' to manage risk and demonstrate to the public and all stakeholders that they are doing so. Controls assurance is described in more detail later in this chapter.

In summary, corporate governance within the NHS is concerned with the non-clinical aspects of healthcare provision, that is ensuring financial and operational success by demonstrating value for money. The link to achieve total governance is that of combining the non-clinical with the clinical aspects of healthcare provision. Perhaps this is the primary influence towards the government's introduction of 'clinical governance' within the NHS.

Activity 2.1: Feedback

Corporate governance is about protecting investors' monies and companies' assets from risks. If these principles are paralleled to the NHS, then corporate governance is about having efficient and effective systems in place to show that money is not being wasted and the services are providing value for money. This is because the NHS is publicly funded via taxation, placing a moral and statutory duty on the management and employees to demonstrate how and where the public money is being spent.

As employees, whether in public or independent sectors, we are governed by contracts of employment, professional regulations and ultimately the civil and criminal laws to provide the best possible services within the given resources. The key word that springs to mind in ensuring corporate governance is *accountability*. Accountability means that you are able to justify your actions, essentially what you do and why you have to do it.

Defining clinical governance

The term clinical governance can be traced to the government's first white paper on health, *The New NHS Modern, Dependable* (DoH 1997) which sets out the government's aims of making the NHS modern and dependable by keeping what has worked in the past and discarding what has failed; for example, the abolition of the internal market that placed finance and activity over clinical quality, leading to fragmentation of services and the ideology of command and control. To resolve these failings the government's philosophy is that of partnerships and collaboration, where innovation is nurtured and staff are valued. The latter is to be achieved by the application of six key principles (see Box 2.2).

Box 2.2 The principles of clinical governance:

1. To re-establish the NHS as a National Service for all patients throughout the country where patients will receive high quality care regardless of age, gender or culture if they are ill or injured.
2. To establish national standards based upon best practices, which will be influenced and delivered locally by the healthcare professionals themselves taking into account the needs of the local population.
3. Collaborative working partnerships between hospital, community services and local authorities, where the patient is the central focus.
4. Ensuring that the services are delivering high quality care and providing value for money.
5. To establish an internal culture where clinical quality is guaranteed for all patients.
6. To enhance public confidence in the NHS.

                                                           Adapted from DoH (1997)

The new structures and systems proposed to achieve the six key principles are:

- A set of national service frameworks to be developed with nationally agreed standards, covering major care areas and disease groups, e.g. cancer services, reducing heart disease, mental health and caring for the older person.
- A new performance framework with a scorecard of quality effectiveness and efficiency measures, rather than the previous cost and activity focus.
- A National Institute for Clinical Excellence (NICE) responsible for the assessment of new technologies and producing robust and authoritative guidelines for the NHS.

- A Commission for Health Improvement (CHi formally known as CHIMP) which will monitor the quality of clinical services at a local level and intervene if necessary to deal with problems.
- A new system of clinical governance which is able to demonstrate, in both primary and secondary care, that systems are in place guaranteeing clinical quality improvements at all levels of healthcare provision.

The structures identified above are all individually directed towards establishing and monitoring the level of clinical quality at individual, organisation, region and national levels; for example, NICE will set standards and guidelines based on the best available evidence accessible nationally for use by individual health professionals. The role of local Trusts and Health Authorities will be to implement these guidelines. The CHi will have the role of monitoring healthcare organisations to ensure that these standards are achieved. Clinical governance according to Donaldson (1998) is viewed as the vehicle to achieve locally the continuous improvements in clinical quality that will aid the government's agenda for modernisation of the NHS, evident from the following statement:

'Chief executives will be expected to ensure there are appropriate local arrangements to give them and the NHS Trust board firm assurances that their responsibilities for quality are being met. This might be through the creation of a Board Sub Committee, led by a named senior consultant, nurse, or other clinical professional, with responsibility for ensuring the internal clinical governance of the organisation.'

(DoH 1997, p. 47)

Clinical governance?

A considerable amount of literature is emerging on the topic of clinical governance, regarding what it is and what it is perceived to be within the various healthcare professions (Scally & Donaldson 1998; Garbett 1998; Harvey 1998; Sealey 1999) as highlighted in Fig. 2.1.

According to Fig. 2.1 clinical governance has similarities in its definition for all healthcare professional groups when translating the government's initial definition of clinical governance. The emerging similarities are associated with having robust systems/frameworks for ensuring that clinical quality exists throughout the entire organisation, where each individual is accountable for their actions. Clinical governance can best be summarised:

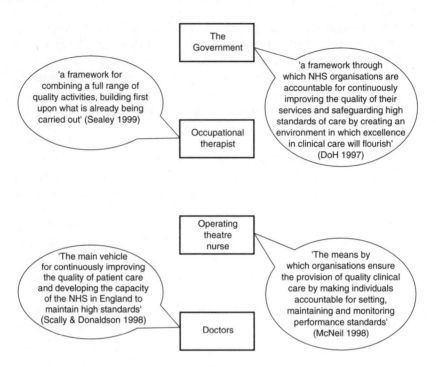

Fig. 2.1   Professional perspectives in defining clinical governance.

'as a protective mechanism for both the public and healthcare professionals, [Fig. 2.2] ensuring that their local hospitals and community trusts are actively developing structures to improve the quality of care in the hope of preventing any reoccurrence of the Bristol Case (R. Smith 1998).'

(McSherry & Haddock 1999)

Clinical governance is 'an umbrella term for all the issues and concepts that clinicians know and foster, including standard setting, risk management, training, reflection and professional development (McSherry & Haddock 1999). Clinical governance is about instilling confidence in both the public and healthcare professionals by providing them with a safe clinical environment in which to accommodate the challenges identified in Chapter 1 which are facing them in the future. In a simple way, clinical governance is about the patients/carers receiving the right care at the right time from the right person in a safe environment. To ensure that clinical governance is successfully implemented throughout the NHS the key components contained within its definition need to be available and

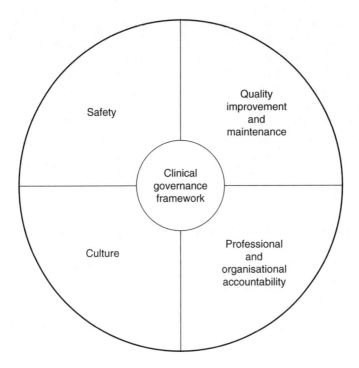

Fig. 2.2   Key components of clinical governance.

achievable throughout the organisation, as the following section will now briefly explain.

The key components of clinical governance

This section introduces the key components of clinical governance and how they relate to individuals, organisations and the wider aspect of the NHS; a more detailed account is offered in Chapter 3.

The definitions of clinical governance provided by DoH (1998), Scally and Donaldson (1998), Sealey (1999), McNeil (1998), RCN (2000) and Roland and Baker (1999) highlight common themes that describe what clinical governance is. These can be summarised into Fig. 2.2.

Figure 2.2 depicts the key components that make up clinical governance, which in turn could be considered as the building blocks for its success for either an individual or a healthcare organisation. For clinical governance to operate effectively the identified components need to be evident and operational. Clinical quality and continuous improvements in healthcare delivery can only be achieved in a culture and environment which supports, values and develops its staff. Likewise individual healthcare professionals need to continuously develop their professional standards whilst operating within the roles and responsibilities aligned to their contract of employment and codes of professional practice. Essentially clinical governance is about providing good clinical care in an environment which places patient and staff safety as a priority.

It is evident from the above description of the authors' interpretations of the DoH (1998), Scally and Donaldson (1998), Sealey (1999) and McNeil (1998) definitions of clinical governance that their primary focus is around clinical practices which no one would disagree with, although within these definitions of clinical governance there appear to be no explicit links to the non-clinical aspects of healthcare which are equally important in proving clinical quality.

Non-clinical services that support clinical governance

Activity 2.2: Non-clinical services that support clinical governance

List the non-clinical services that support healthcare professionals in executing clinical governance successfully.

Read on and compare your findings with those in the Feedback box towards the end of the chapter.

When providing care in a busy and stressful clinical setting it is easy to forget all those other supporting services that are perhaps taken for granted when we provide our services; for example, a simple case of a General Practitioner referring a patient to a consultant for a clinical opinion. This involves the letter from the GP, perhaps dictated for their clerical staff to process, which may be received by the medical records staff or consultant secretaries who in turn arrange an outpatient appointment and inform the patient. The patient subsequently attends the outpatient department to be seen by the consultant. For this to happen effectively, much work is done behind the scenes that involves the following groups of personnel: estate staffs in maintaining the safety of the building and mains services; domestics in maintaining the cleanliness and hygiene standards; and a range of supporting services to enable the operational and clinical staff to perform their duties, such as personnel, finance and information services. Clinical governance cannot be operationalised without the non-clinical supporting services, as depicted by the simple example above. This example demonstrates the links between non-clinical supporting activity and clinical governance. Clinical governance cannot be successfully implemented without the support of the non-clinical aspects of healthcare delivery. As most health professionals are fully aware, healthcare provision and delivery is complex in nature. Successful healthcare delivery is

dependent on good teamwork, effective leadership and sound management in drawing together the non-clinical and clinical aspects of governance. Basically neither can work effectively without the other, as outlined
in Fig. 2.3.

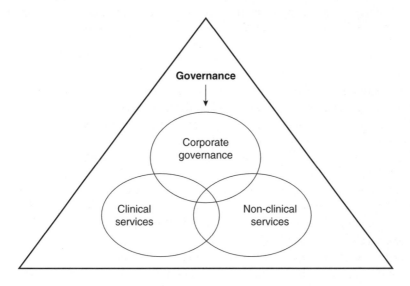

Fig. 2.3 Healthcare governance in the NHS.

Figure 2.3 highlights the role of healthcare governance in uniting the
three elements of health service governance: corporate (management),
clinical governance (clinical practice) and the non-clinical supporting
services. Whilst there has been much attention directed towards establishing good managerial and clinical practices based on sound evidence in
ensuring clinical quality, it would appear that ensuring quality associated
with the non-clinical supporting services such as those outlined in Activity
2.2 was not given equal status. To address this imbalance it is important to
know that the government has introduced guidelines and standards for the
NHS to assure quality in these parts of the organisation. This is to be
achieved by the introduction of 'controls assurance' (NHS Executive
1999).

Controls assurance

The Health Service Circular 1999/123 describes controls assurance as 'A
holistic concept based on best governance practice' (NHS Executive 1999,

p. 2). This approach is reinforced and enhanced by Emslie who defines controls assurance as:

> 'a process, built on best governance practice, by which NHS organi-sations demonstrate that they are doing their reasonable best to manage themselves so as to meet their objectives and protect patients, staff, visitors, and other stakeholders against risks of all kinds.'

> (Emslie 2001, p. 1)

The difficulty for many healthcare organisations and individuals is in conceptualising and implementing healthcare governance because they see each component, such as clinical governance, corporate governance and controls assurance, as separate and unrelated entities. The authors accept that many healthcare professionals view the components of healthcare governance in isolation, but we would argue that in practice this is usually not the case. For example, the routine administration of either an intra-venous or intramuscular injection involves many clinical and non-clinical healthcare professionals and systems and processes to work efficiently and effectively. Some healthcare professionals only see their part of the overall systems and process(es), such as the preparation and administration. But what happens if the medication and equipment are not available or the 'sharps' are not disposed of safely? This simple illustration demonstrates that healthcare governance is truly a holistic concept that unifies the three components of clinical, non-clinical and corporate governance. Controls assurance is the vehicle that enables each organisation to demonstrate that their systems and processes for assuring healthcare governance are both efficient and effective.

Emslie (2001) provides a model linking corporate (Trust) objectives with providing assurance to their stakeholders of quality healthcare, highlighting the importance of accountability, processes, capability and outcomes, of which each element is continuously monitored and reviewed, and where lessons are learnt, practices improved and risks minimised. Essentially this model can be applied to individuals, teams and organisa-tions. Controls assurance is concerned with methods that enable health-care organisations to provide evidence that they are doing their 'reasonable best' to manage risk and demonstrate to the public and all stakeholders that they are doing so. The main principle underpinning controls assurance is that of collaborative working, thus ensuring that risks are minimised and where identified are managed appropriately (McSherry & Pearce 2000; Emslie 2001).

Within the Health Service Circular HSC 1999/123 chief executives were advised to appoint an executive director to assume responsibility for the implementation of controls assurance, thus making an individual the accountable officer to parliament. The designated person is charged with reviewing the circular and guidance. Chief executives are responsible for informing the National Controls Assurance Project Manager who is the designated person for their organisation.

The HSC 1999/123 led to the development of 18 standards covering the non-clinical and some clinical aspects of service delivery, such as infection control, health and safety and waste management. The standards were released on 22 November 1999 at the NHS Controls Assurance Conference which 'forms the basis of a self-assessment exercise to be undertaken by all NHS trusts and health authorities this year, leading up to an assurance statement to be signed by chief executives on behalf of boards in their 1999–2000 annual report' (Hopkins 2000, p. 22). In essence controls assurance completes the governance picture by linking the corporate, clinical and non-clinical elements of governance.

More information on controls assurance can be found at the NHS Controls Assurance Team's website at www.open.gov.uk/doh/risk-man.htm, or by reading McSherry and Pearce (2000), NHS Executive (1999) and Hopkins (2000). It is clear from Fig. 2.1 that the key elements of governance all have potential benefits to improve the quality of care that can be further enhanced when these components work in harmony.

Potential advantages and disadvantages of governance in the NHS for organisations and individuals

The potential advantages and disadvantages of introducing governance into the NHS are vast. Principally clinical governance could be seen as the primary vehicle for the 'delivery of the quality agenda through a model of shared decision making' (Garland 1998, p. 28). Essentially health service governance is about the development of genuine collaborative working partnerships between employees and employers in facilitating an environment in which clinical care will flourish (S. Smith 1998). The potential advantages and disadvantages of clinical governance are outlined in Table 2.1.

The main points of the table can be summarised as: there are some similarities and differences for NHS organisations, professional staff, and the public; assuring quality and safety are the common benefits; a lack of time and resources could be a barrier to successful implementation.

Table 2.1 Potential advantages and disadvantages of clinical governance.

	Organisations	Professionals	Public
Advantages	• Offers a strategic direction for trusts • Provides a mechanism for quality control, assurance and improvement • Encourages frameworks and systems to be developed • Clarifies accountability • Aligns staff to the organisation's needs • Encourages collaborative working • Reduces and manages risks • Facilitates cultural change • Encourages new and innovative practices • Pertinacity to reduce litigation • Universal access to services and equity of services	• Continuing professional development, learning from mistakes • Staff are valued • Improved open and honest working relationships • Reduced risk and improved safety • Greater staff involvement • Enhanced collaboration	• Provides quality assurance • Greater access to information on clinical performance • Reduced risks • Increased satisfaction • More involvement • Equity of access
Disadvantages	• Time • Costs/resources • Could be seen as a policing mechanism • Potential to reduce innovation • Openness to criticism • Long term strategy • Potential of increased litigation costs	• More demands placed on busy people • Lack of knowledge and skills • Raised unrealistic expectations	• Lack of understanding • Unreal expectations of the NHS

Note: This is by no means an exhaustive list and is not placed in any order of priority.

Activity 2.2 Feedback

Non-clinical services that support the implementation of clinical governance:

- Finance
- Personnel (human resources)
- Estates: building, electrical and mechanical services
- Catering
- Domestic services
- Information technology
- Administration and clerical services
- Medical records
- Library services

Note: This is by no means an exhaustive list and is not placed in any order of priority.

Conclusion

In conclusion, clinical governance is a highly complex and multifaceted concept dependent upon successful integration of corporate governance and controls assurance. The successful integration of these three elements within any healthcare organisation we believe could result in the achievement of 'healthcare governance'. Healthcare governance is about establishing frameworks for sustaining and improving clinical quality which can only take place when the organisational infrastructures support the overall aims of corporate, clinical and non-clinical aspects of governance.

Garside (1999) reinforces our term 'healthcare governance' by suggesting that clinical governance is 'the opportunity to change systems – to pull together different components and strands from the clinical and managerial worlds to improve things for patients'. The challenge for the NHS is in 'converging' all of the governance components under a single umbrella which all healthcare professionals can access, understand, implement and evaluate at a level most suited to their roles and responsibilities in the attempt to minimise risks. Convergence has already been recognised by the DoH:

> 'We are committed to achieving a fully integrated approach to governance where clinical and corporate governance sits side by side – clinical governance focusing on continuous improvements in quality and corporate governance focusing on having the necessary systems in place to minimise risk.'

(Reeves 2001, p. 1)

The Health Service Circular 2001/005 (NHS Executive 2001) provides advice and guidance together with a timetable for this to occur within the NHS by 2005.

To develop your understandings about clinical governance the key components will be examined in detail in Chapter 3.

KEY POINTS

- **Corporate governance**

Corporate governance in general is about protecting investors' monies and companies' assets from risks. Likewise corporate governance in the NHS is about ensuring that public monies have not been wasted in healthcare delivery.

- **Clinical governance**

Clinical governance is a framework for the continual improvement of patient care by minimising clinical risks and continuing the development of organisations and staff.

- **Controls assurance**

Controls assurance is about assuring quality within healthcare organisations for the non-clinical supporting services such as health and safety and clinical waste management.

- **Healthcare governance**

Healthcare governance is the harmonisation of corporate governance, clinical governance and controls assurance.

RECOMMENDED READING

Hopkins, B. (2000) National Controls Assurance Conference. *Health Care Risk Report*, 6(3) 22–24.

NHS Executive (1999) *Health Services Circular 1999/123 Governance in the New NHS: Controls Assurance Statements 1999/2000: Risk Management and Organizational Controls*. DoH, London.

Roland, M. & Baker, R. (1999) *Clinical Governance practical guide for primary care teams*. The National Primary Care Research and Development Centre, University of Manchester and University of Leicester.

RCN (2000) *Clinical Governance: How nurses can get involved*. Royal College of Nursing, London.

Smith, S. (1998) Model Behaviour. *Nursing Management*, 5(6) 19–24.

USEFUL WEBSITES

Controls Assurance Support Unit: www.casu.org.uk
DoH Controls Assurance: www.doh.gov.uk/riskman.htm

References

Chua-Eoan, H. (1995) Cover: Leeson Destroys Barings: Going for Broke. http://www.time.com/time/magazine/archive/1995/950313/950313.cover.html

DoH (1994) *Corporate Governance in the NHS, Code of Conduct, Code of Accountability*. The Stationery Office, London.

DoH (1997) *The New NHS Modern and Dependable*. The Stationery Office, London.

DoH (1998) *A First Class Service: Quality in the new NHS*. The Stationery Office, London.

Donaldson, L. J. (1998) Clinical governance: quality improvement as a duty, not a choice. *Healthcare Quality*, 4 (3) 7–9.

Emslie, S. (2001) Controls assurance in the National Health Service in England – the final piece of the corporate governance jigsaw. *Corporate Governance*, 12, March, Abg Professional Information, London.

Garbett, R. (1998) Clinical Governance? *Nursing Times Learning Centre*, 12 (7) 15.

Garland, G. (1998) Governance. *Nursing Management*, 5 (6) 28–31.

Garside, P. (1999) Book review. Clinical Governance: Making it happen (eds M. Lugon & J. Secker-Walker, RSM Press, London). *BMJ*, 318, 881.

Harvey, G. (1998) Improving patient care. *RCN Magazine*, Autumn.

Hopkins, B. (2000) National Controls Assurance Conference. *Health Care Risk Report*, 6 (3) 22–24.

McNeil, J. (1998) Clinical governance: The whys, whats, and hows for theatre practitioners. *British Journal of Theatre Nursing*, 9 (5) 208–216.

McSherry, R. & Haddock, J. (1999) *Evidence based health care: Its place within clinical governance. British Journal of Nursing*, 8 (2) 113–117.

McSherry, R. & Pearce, P. K. (2000) Interpreting the new controls guidelines. *Health Care Risk Report*, 6(3) 19–21.

NHS Executive (1999) *Health Service Circular 1999/123 Governance in the New NHS: Controls Assurance Statements 1999/2000: Risk Management and Organizational Controls*. DoH, London.

NHS Executive (2001) *Health Service Circular 2001/005 'Controls Assurance Statements 2000/2001 and Establishment of The Controls Assurance Support Unit*. DoH, London.

RCN (2000) *Clinical Governance: How nurses can get involved*. Royal College of Nursing, London.

Reeves, C. (2001) Letter: *Governance in the NHS*. NHS Executive, Leeds.

Roland, M. & Baker, R. (1999) *Clinical Governance practical guide for primary care teams*. The National Primary Care Research and Development Centre, University of Manchester and University of Leicester.

Scally, G. & Donaldson, L. J. (1998), Clinical governance and the drive for quality improvement in the new NHS in England. *BMJ*, 317, 4 July.

Sealey, C. (1999) Clinical Governance: An Information Guide for Occupational Therapists. *British Journal of Occupational Therapy*, 62 (6).

Smith, R. (1998a) All changed, changed utterly: British Medicine will be transformed by the Bristol Case. *BMJ*, 316, 1917–18.

Smith, S. (1998b) Model behaviour. *Nursing Management*, 5 (6) 19–24.

Chapter 3

A Guide to Clinical Governance

Rob McSherry and Paddy Pearce

Introduction

The previous chapters looked at the contributing factors that led to the introduction of clinical governance, and what clinical governance is. This chapter builds on the previous chapter by exploring and explaining in detail the key components of clinical governance by the application and modification of McSherry and Haddock's (1999) framework and by referring to the government's NHS Executive circulars on clinical governance and its associated components.

The key components of clinical governance

As outlined in Chapter 2, clinical governance has several themes associated with its definition: quality improvements and maintenance, professional accountability, creating and maintaining a safe environment for patients and staff along with establishing an honest and open culture that encourages and responds to staff and public opinion – key themes for all healthcare organisations and individuals to develop in pursuit of clinical excellence.

The issue facing many healthcare organisations and individual health professionals is not in distinguishing the key themes associated with clinical governance, because we all want to practise in a clinical environment that proactively develops its staff and services in order to enhance the standards and quality of care, treatments or interventions. The concerns expressed by many healthcare professionals focus on answering the questions of implementing clinical governance for organisations and individuals as highlighted in Box 3.1.

Describing the key components of clinical governance

Box 3.1 Questions associated with describing the key components of clinical governance

- What are the key components of clinical governance?
- Is clinical governance only an organisational concern?
- How do you implement a system of clinical governance?
- Can a clinical governance framework be developed for individual health-care professionals to use in pursuit of clinical excellence?

Box 3.1 is not an exhaustive list of questions raised by healthcare professionals in highlighting the practicalities of developing and implementing a system of clinical governance. Box 3.1 demonstrates staff's concerns and confusions over what clinical governance has to offer at an organisational, team and individual level in improving the quality and standards of care. Essentially clinical governance is the term used to focus individual and organisational attentions back to quality: 'So that quality is at the core, both of their responsibilities as organisations and of each of their staff as individual professionals' (DoH 1997a, p. 47). The government's quote on clinical governance clearly responds to the questions raised in Box 3.1 by suggesting that both individual healthcare professionals and their organisations are to work within the framework of clinical governance.

Activity 3.1: Key components of clinical governance

In Chapter 2 we identified how clinical governance is about promoting, maintaining and evaluating best practices. To achieve clinical excellence at an individual and organisational level, what systems or infrastructures do you feel should be in place to achieve this goal?

Write down your responses on a sheet of paper and then read on and compare your findings with those at the end of the chapter.

Before outlining the key components of clinical governance it is essential to describe the relationship between the healthcare organisation and the achievement of quality care.

Healthcare organisations and the achievement of quality care

Clinical excellence will flourish in an organisation that proactively responds to incidents, complaints or suggestions by the public or staff regarding their experience of providing or receiving nursing care, treatments or interventions from healthcare professionals or service users. Scally and Donaldson (1998) develop the idea of quality dependence and organisational stability/instability in detail by offering an illustration that describes the variations in the quality of health by focusing on low and high quality practices. A bell curve is offered with low quality at one end and high quality at the other. Where low or poor quality is experienced, potential problems could exist in the form of untoward incidents and increased complaints; the aim is for healthcare organisations to shift changes in practice from the centre or mean towards the high quality. Whilst the Scally and Donaldson (1998) illustration outlining the variations in the quality of health organisations is a useful way of viewing the standards of quality, it is not without its limitations. For example, how does an organisation establish the mean or best practices for a certain service? How does the organisation or individual know that the standards of practice are of high or low quality?

To address some of the above limitations and to further build on Scally and Donaldson's (1998) work it is important to demonstrate the link between proactive and reactionary organisational management in achieving clinical excellence, and its association with implementing a clinical governance framework as depicted in Fig. 3.1.

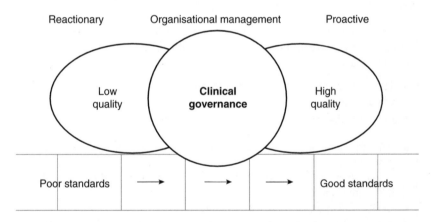

Fig. 3.1   Clinical excellence and its association with organisational management styles.

It is clear from Fig. 3.1 that a system of clinical governance will only be achieved where a balance between reactionary and proactive management exists within the healthcare organisation; this will hopefully result in the continued provision of medium to high quality care. To achieve high quality care it is essential that the right culture and clinical environments and services are created, and this depends on nurturing a proactive approach to management. That is not to say reactionary management is ineffective, because there may be occasions when this type of approach is advocated. To create an open culture that positively seeks and responds to criticisms and compliments will take time, but it is the preferred style advocated within the clinical governance frameworks.

So what are the qualities required by an organisation to become more proactive in nature? Scally and Donaldson (1998) and Donaldson & Muir Gray (1998) indicate that quality improvements are dependent on having an:

> 'organisation-wide approach to quality improvement with emphasis on preventing adverse outcomes through simplification and improving the process of care. Leadership and commitment from the top of the organisation, team work, consumer focus, and good data are also important.'

> (Scally & Donaldson 1998, p. 62)

These are key attributes inferred by having a proactive management approach.

The white paper *The New NHS Modern, Dependable* (DoH 1997a) describes how a quality organisation can be achieved by proactively ensuring that the ten attributes and processes shown in Box 3.2 are present.

Box 3.2 Key attributes associated with promotion of a quality organisation

- There is an integrated approach to quality improvement throughout the whole organisation.
- Leadership skills are developed in line with professional and clinical needs.
- Infrastructures exist that foster the development of evidence based practices.
- Innovations are valued and good practices are shared within and without the organisation.
- Clinical risk management systems are in place.
- There is a proactive approach to reporting and dealing with and learning from untoward incidents.
- Complaints are taken seriously and actions taken to prevent any recurrence.
- Ensuring that poor clinical performance is recognised thus preventing potential harm to patients or staff.
- Practice and professional development is aligned and integral to clinical governance frameworks.
- Clinical data is of the best quality and can be used effectively to monitor patient care and clinical outcomes.

Adapted from (DoH 1997a)

It is evident from Box 3.2 that the establishment of a proactive organisational culture is dependent on the development of 'effective channels of communication between healthcare professionals' (McSherry & Haddock 1999) and infrastructures such as education, training, research and access to high quality information in supporting staff in their pursuit of clinical excellence. Essentially, 'successful quality improvement demands major cultural change – but that change cannot simply be imposed, as it entails a significant shift in the way that people think and behave' (Walshe *et al.* 2000, p. 1). The question that often remains unanswered in much of the literature reviewed by the authors is, how do you achieve successful culture change(s)?

Figure 3.1 demonstrates how a proactive management style is the best way to promote an honest and open culture which can and will only be achieved through strong leadership and commitment to genuine quality improvement. This approach to management, of openly encouraging a shared ownership for the active development, implementation and evaluation of the infrastructures associated with clinical governance, is the key to success. Involvement of staff from all levels within and without the organisation needs to be carefully considered. Without the involvement and cooperation of clinical staff, clinical governance will not make a difference to patient care.

A possible approach for encouraging positive cultural shifts or changes in attitudes is that offered by McSherry & Haddock (1999) in highlighting the key components and structures of evidence based practice (see Fig. 3.2).

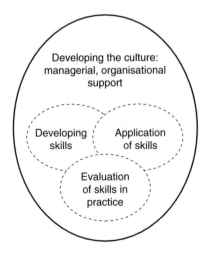

Fig. 3.2 Promoting a culture for evidence based practice within clinical governance. (*Reproduced with kind permission from Mark Allen Publishing Ltd.*)

Figure 3.2 describes how the development of the staff's culture is paramount if successful implementation of evidence based practice in relation to clinical governance is to be achieved. The key components are the development, application and evaluation of practices that can be used at organisational and individual levels.

The same approach could be transferred to the development of clinical governance in that the correct organisational culture needs to be established whilst the infrastructures are being developed and implemented. The starting point for healthcare organisations to successfully implement clinical governance is to review the white papers (DoH 1997a, 1998) and Department of Health guidance documents, NHS Circular 1999/065 (NHS Executive 1999a), on clinical governance with reference to local internal organisational structures and policies.

It is evident from the information presented thus far, that clinical governance is a highly complex system containing and involving many themes and management and organisational processes in the pursuit of individual and organisational clinical quality. What remains to be described and discussed is how to ensure that clinical governance becomes a reality for all practising healthcare professionals, NHS personnel and healthcare organisations.

Upon reading the NHS Circular 1999/065 and the literature by Edwards and Packham (1999), McSherry and Haddock (1999) and Donaldson (2000), several key themes emerge that encompass the key elements of clinical governance (Fig. 3.3). It is evident from Fig. 3.3 that risk management, performance management, quality improvement, information and accountability are central to the delivery of clinical governance. This will now be outlined in more detail.

Risk management

Risk management simply means practising safely: 'It aims to develop good practice and reduce the occurrence of harmful or adverse incidents' (RCN 2000 p. 19). The concept of risk management is about the reduction of clinical and non-clinical risks associated with healthcare. In the past, risk management focused on the financial areas of healthcare. It is important to remember when exploring the notion of risk that the following definitions of risk could be applied to either the clinical or non-clinical aspects of healthcare:

- A variation in the outcomes that could occur over a specified period in a given situation (Williams & Heins 1976).
- The possibility of incurring misfortune or loss (Collins 1985)
- The chance or possibility of bad outcome (Wilson & Tingle 1999).

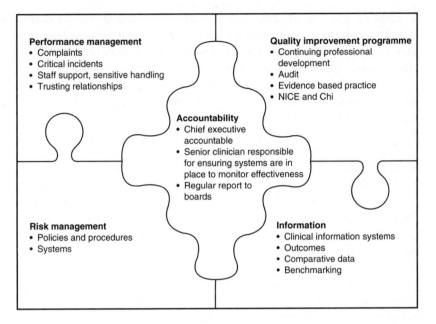

Performance management
- Complaints
- Critical incidents
- Staff support, sensitive handling
- Trusting relationships

Quality improvement programme
- Continuing professional development
- Audit
- Evidence based practice
- NICE and Chi

Accountability
- Chief executive accountable
- Senior clinician responsible for ensuring systems are in place to monitor effectiveness
- Regular report to boards

Risk management
- Policies and procedures
- Systems

Information
- Clinical information systems
- Outcomes
- Comparative data
- Benchmarking

Fig. 3.3 Key components of clinical governance. (Modified from the McSherry & Haddock (1999) template outlining clinical governance.)

Healthcare governance is about the management of 'risk' regardless of its origins within the corporate systems and processes. Some healthcare professionals, teams and organisations tend to view 'risk' in relation to their own position and profession and not in a holistic manner; this may result in only partial reductions and minimisations of a given risk, which may be seen only as a clinical risk. Clinical risk is defined as 'a clinical error to be at variance from intended treatment, care, therapeutic intervention or diagnostic result; there may be an untoward outcome or not' (Wilson & Tingle 1999, p. 71). This notion is evidenced in the following example. Several patients in a specific clinical area develop wound infections resulting in extended lengths of stay, patient discomfort and increased workload and costs for staff working in that organisation. If this situation was identified by a clinician as a professional issue only, they might identify the clinical risk but fail to consider the broader issues surrounding this situation, such as ward cleanliness, adherence to infection control policies and procedures, addressing education and training and overall considerations of resource allocation and finance.

Risk management is mainly 'concerned with harnessing the information and expertise of individuals within the organisation and translating that with their help into positive action which will reduce loss of life, financial loss, loss of staff availability, loss of the availability of buildings or equipment and loss of reputation' (DoH 1994). Within the context of healthcare governance the identification and management of risks should be viewed in a holistic way associated with the clinical, environmental and operational aspects of the incident, situation or event.

However, the most important aspect, that of clinical quality, was underdeveloped (DoH 2000). This philosophy over the past several years has changed significantly. It would seem that since the lifting of crown immunity in 1995, where central government was responsible for the payment of clinical negligence claims for all NHS organisations, a shift in responsibility to the individual NHS organisations has occurred for the settlement of such claims. This change in policy made NHS organisations seriously consider how their organisation and staff were managing risks. In response to the lifting of crown immunity, NHS Trusts realised the need to address this issue of protecting themselves from the pursuit of clinical negligence claims which would have to be financed from their annual budgets.

The lifting of crown immunity led to the establishment of the Clinical Negligence Scheme for Trusts (CNST) in 1995. The basic principle of the scheme is similar to a personal, household or car insurance where you pay your premiums and obtain discounts for no-claims. With CNST you pay your premiums based on the size of your hospital, its specialties, and on your claims history, and you receive discount for minimising and managing clinical risks. The level of discount is associated with achieving compliance with standards ranging from level one to three. The higher the level of accreditation against the required standards, the greater the discount. Essentially the CNST is a pooling scheme for its members where, should a huge negligence claim be made against a Trust, the scheme would pay out the settlement after the Trust had paid its excess (Mayatt 1995).

The standards are concerned with having:

- A clinical risk strategy.
- An identified executive director responsible for the management of clinical risk.
- A system for reporting, monitoring and evaluating clinical incidence and near misses (i.e. a potentially harmful incident that could have had adverse consequences for a patient/carer).
- A major clinical incident policy, e.g. to address an infectious disease outbreak or medical equipment failure.
- A system for complaints reporting, monitoring and actioning.
- Consent and advice policies available, i.e. Patients are informed of the risks and benefits of a procedure from an individual capable of doing that procedure.
- Policies for the recording, storing and auditing of all patient records.

- Systems for induction training and the ongoing development of professional competence.
- Clinical standards for the promotion of clinical quality pertinent to specialty groups, e.g. maternity, mental health and ambulance.

The CNST offers a framework to minimise and manage clinical risks in the pursuit of clinical excellence. Initially CNST was intended to reduce financial risks: 'a large settlement or a series of sizable settlements could significantly impinge upon the overall financial position of a Trust' (Mayatt 1995, p. 2). Today CNST is a voluntary organisation administered by the NHS Litigation Authority, that can support the clinical risk aspect of clinical governance. CNST offers a framework for the management of clinical risk, although there continues to be room for ongoing development and improving the clinical risk infrastructures as alluded to by the Chief Medical Officer (DoH 2000). An example of improved clinical risk infrastructures could be the establishment of a national incident reporting system to detect potential clinical risks for all NHS organisations at an early stage. This approach to the management of risks was highlighted in *An Organisation with a Memory* (DoH 2000) and how it will be actioned via *Building a Safer NHS for Patents: Implementing an Organisation with a Memory* (DoH 2001).

It is important to mention here that whilst the CNST standards have done much to advance risk management and reduce clinical risks, a need for a holistic management of 'risk' has been introduced via the controls assurance standards (www.doh.gov/riskman.htm) which further enhance a whole systems approach towards risk management within the NHS in England. These are standards to which all healthcare organisations must adhere.

Managing performance

The DoH (1997a) reforms of the NHS provided a performance assessment framework that supports the drive for higher quality standards by ensuring that performance assessment is focused on the delivery of effective, appropriate and timely health services which meet local needs (DoH 1997a, p. 63).

Within the clinical governance framework the management of poor performance of either devices or personnel is imperative in reducing clinical failures. As highlighted earlier in this chapter, management styles play an important part in how people perform. In addition to having a proactive management style and an honest and open culture which encourages staff and the public to express ideas or concerns, how can an organisation detect, promote and deal with good or poor performance?

It is acknowledged within the literature (RCN 2000; DoH 2000) that the delivery of healthcare involves many complex processes involving many individuals to provide the best service to the public. With this in mind it is easier to apportion blame to individuals rather than the systems when things go wrong. This is because for many organisations reviewing systems is time consuming and costly, and for some organisations it is about establishing where to start. The easy option is to blame the individual when things go wrong, but this reactionary approach is not beneficial to preventing recurrence of the situation. What is needed is a review of the systems and processes associated with the incident, and to be honest and open with the findings. This proactive approach to dealing with incidents or complaints involving individuals, teams or processes requires a major cultural shift, as eloquently described by the Royal College of Nursing:

'A culture that encourages open discussion and reflection on practice allows staff to learn from their experiences. This includes both celebrating what is done well and learning from what is done less well. However, if an organisation is going to encourage clinicians to report incidents and learn from mistakes, it must develop a blame free culture, rather than one that revolves around disciplinary procedures.'

(RCN 2000, p. 8)

It is evident from the RCN's definition that performance management in healthcare services needs to be reorganised to deal with good and poor performances, as this has not been the case in the past. Achieving this goal is about developing simple but effective systems and processes that capture performances of individuals, teams, organisations and devices which work well and not so well. The overall aim of this type of performance management is to establish, share and learn from the experiences of others.

Activity 3.2: Performance management

Write down what you think influences the performance of an individual, team or organisation, along with the systems and processes that should be developed in an organisation to assist in dealing with good or poor performance.

Compare your responses with those in the Feedback box at the end of the chapter.

We believe two main factors influence performance management in the NHS: the perceived experiences of the public and the organisation's philosophical approach to performance. Figure 3.4 provides a framework outlining the various components associated with performance management, of which more is explained below.

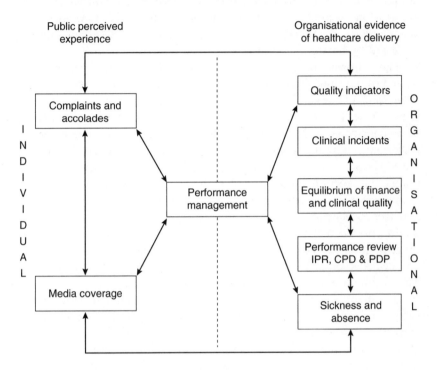

Fig. 3.4 Framework for performance management.

Figure 3.4 shows how performance management is about dealing with good and not so good performance. It is clear that the public's view is based upon individuals' experience of, or the media coverage of, the services or a combination of both. Often 'all that is good in healthcare is regarded by the public as being attributable to doctors and nurses, while all that is bad is the fault of managers and their political masters' (Baker 1998, p. 137). The quote by Baker is plausible and in most cases true, but for performance management to operate effectively within the context of clinical governance frameworks, this conception needs to be changed. Baker's quote seems to suggest that the public and perhaps many health service staff fail to understand that performance depends on uniting the non-clinical infrastructures with the clinical, along with the processes and systems associated with each. Poor performance can often be the result of systems and process failure rather than individuals. Systems are only as good as the design; if this is ineffective then so is the information or care given as a result. To develop good performance management systems within the context of clinical governance, Acute and Community Trusts, Primary Care Trusts or Health Authority boards need to embrace a philosophy that proactively encourages the concept of performance management. In a simple way they need to be able to answer two questions: What are we doing? How well are we doing it? These can only be answered by having the appropriate systems in place to collect and disseminate information associated with good and not so good performance related to the clinical and non-clinical aspects of healthcare service.

Figure 3.4 shows that there are several systems and processes that need to be in place to provide information on performance. Performance needs to be considered in line with a whole systems approach, where clinical performance and non-clinical performance are seen as equal. In the past the NHS has tended to focus on financial performance and activity, i.e. the number of patient treatments and length of waiting lists. This information is important and needs to be collected; however, it does not provide managers or the public with any information about the quality of care and services provided or indeed how individuals or systems are performing. A range of quality indicators need to be developed that provide information and evidence on either individual, team or organisational performance. These systems and associated processes need to capture activity from a variety of sources, i.e. organisational, team and individual performance such as pressure sore prevalence and hospital acquired infections. If we apply these examples to Fig. 3.4 it is evident how systems such as clinical incident reporting, complaints and accolades monitoring, financial and quality reporting, performance reviews and the recording of sickness and absence, can demonstrate the overall performance of individuals, teams and the organisation. This is because each part of the performance management system includes reviewing and acting on the information given in demonstrating good or not so good practice, which can be highlighted through pooling information gathered from several systems and processes such as the following.

Clinical incident reporting
Clinical incident reporting is required for staff and patients in highlighting any areas where an individual or organisation fails to deliver the appropriate standard of care. Incident reporting offers a framework for the detection of untoward incidents and near misses, which enables action to be taken, lessons to be learnt, practices to be reviewed and information to be shared to prevent any recurrence.

Individual performance review
Individual performance review (IPR) should encourage staff to express

and report any concerns about their own individual practices so that continued improvements can be made in the delivery of services and in promoting safe practice. Following an IPR an individual professional or personal development plan should be written and agreed by the parties to enable the individual and department to develop their practices in line with the overall direction of the employing organisation (Martin 2000).

Complaints and accolades monitoring
Complaints and accolades monitoring elicits trends and patterns in care delivery, enabling the most appropriate action to be taken or indeed to celebrate areas of good performance.

Sickness and absence monitoring
Sickness and absence monitoring enables either the individual, teams or organisation to evaluate the well-being of personnel and can be used to help explain areas of poor performance, e.g. rising numbers of clinical complaints in a ward area because of staff shortages due to sickness and absence.

In summary, performance management is about the integration and utilisation of data and information obtained from services often viewed with negative connotations, such as clinical incident reporting, complaints and clinical audit. However, these systems and processes should be viewed positively, because they often demonstrate the existence of quality services and standards of practice. Performance management is about the integration of the various systems and sources of information in highlighting the overall quality status of the organisation (Garland 1998).

Quality improvement

'Clinical governance' is about assuring sustainable continuous quality improvement, which can only be achieved by the determined and conscious efforts of the clinical and non-clinical staff who have the appropriate support of their organisation to deliver best practice. To obtain improvements in quality systems there needs to be in place appropriate support to facilitate individuals and organisations in the pursuit of clinical excellence (NHS Executive 1999a). Continuous quality improvement is the route to clinical excellence. Clinical excellence can only be achieved by having efficient and effective systems of communication with staff and patients and where infrastructures are established that proactively seek to develop, maintain and monitor the standards and quality of care provided by the organisation and individuals themselves. The words 'vigilant' and 'surveillance' come to mind in ensuring that the term clinical governance becomes an integral part of all daily practices. Figure 3.5 highlights how clinical excellence can be achieved by having an organisation that continually seeks to improve its standards and practices by having integrated systems of clinical risk management, clinical audit, and practices based on sound evidence which form the basis of staff development.

It becomes apparent from Fig 3.5 that quality improvement is based around the following systems and processes.

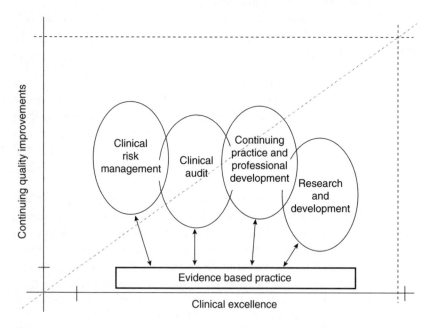

Fig. 3.5   Continuous quality improvement: the route to clinical excellence.

Clinical risk management and audit

As outlined previously in this chapter, risk management is about the development of robust systems which assist staff in establishing efficient and effective standards of care against local, national or international standards, in an attempt to minimise risks.

Clinical audit is defined as the systematic and critical review of systems and processes of care, a method which is essential to compare performance against evidence based standards, for example compliance with National Institute for Clinical Excellence (NICE) guidelines. NICE has been responsible for the appraisal and assessment of new and existing technologies and for producing guidelines for the NHS. Clinical audit is the tool to measure compliance of treatment, interventions or care offered to patients, and the resulting effectiveness on patient care. Areas of poor practice or potential risk should be highlighted so that standards or local policies and guidelines can be written to prevent incidents or harm to patients.

Continued practice and professional development

To ensure that an organisation and staff deliver a high quality service they need to have sound knowledge and well developed skills and competencies to perform their roles efficiently and effectively. Lifelong learning and continuing professional development (CPD) should be seen as an ongoing process in ensuring that practices are the most effective and up to date. The term CPD was originally mentioned in the government's white papers (DoH 1997a, 1998) where the government set out its long-term goal of modernising the NHS, with the key focus for change centred on quality improvements. In order to achieve this, health care organisations must have robust systems and processes to ensure the continued professional development of all their employees.

CPD is defined as:

'A process of lifelong learning for all individuals and teams which meets the needs of patients and delivers the health outcomes and healthcare priorities of the NHS and which enables professionals to expand and fulfil their potential.'

(DoH 1998, p. 42)

CPD should be seen as the beginning of a process of developing a culture of lifelong learning for all staff. To develop a robust system and process for the delivery of CPD local ownership is essential. We do recognise that this is a long-term objective, will take several years to achieve and requires the backing from the chairs and chief executives of healthcare organisations because they have a key role to play in ensuring CPD via collaboration and communication between managers, human resources, nursing and medical education committees, and in ensuring that the educational aspect of CPD meets their organisation's and professional staff's requirements. CPD is for all parts of the NHS; with the increasingly competitive labour market the NHS needs to pay attention to the development of managers and information technology personnel in order to ensure access to current information in supporting the development of their employees and services. To facilitate the development of a system for CPD within a healthcare organisation or team or for individuals, it is imperative to action the points outlined in the Health Service Circular 1999/154 *Continuing Professional Development: Quality in The New*

NHS (NHS Executive 1999b). To illustrate how this can be achieved, the following example is taken from Pearce & McSherry (2000).

Implementing continuing professional development within an NHS Trust

In order to implement HSC 1999/154 within the NHS, individual organisations need to adopt a focused approach to ensure the delivery of high quality care, an approach that could be enhanced by the development of robust CPD. In applying this principle the concept of 'management' by objectives could be introduced. This style of managing CPD enables the Trust to anticipate and highlight important issues relevant to the needs of their healthcare population. Corporate objectives are set prior to the start of the financial year, which are specific to the core elements of the Trust's business plan. From these core objectives, subobjectives for clinical and general managers are established and linked to the personal development plans (PDP) for their staff. A PDP is linked to the individual's annual performance appraisal where the employee and manager review the year's progress and assess strengths, weaknesses, opportunities and threats (SWOT analysis), jointly agreeing an individual plan for the next twelve months with a six-monthly review. This approach enables the Trust to systematically identify the important national, regional and local issues to inform a coherent and coordinated strategy in achieving the objectives. This approach to CPD ensures that the Trust is working collaboratively as a team. Figure 3.6 illustrates a model for the CPD processes.

CPD will be discussed in more detail in Chapter 4, but it is worth noting here that CPD is a key element of the Investors in People Award which many healthcare organisations and teams aspire to (for more information on this award visit the website http:www.Iip.co.uk). It is evident from the above information that CPD and lifelong learning are integral aspects of the clinical governance framework and can only be achieved by mutual collaboration, respect, openness and honesty between employees and employers about how the individual and the organisation are performing. Successful implementation depends on adequate resourcing and genuine commitment from all parties involved, i.e. from the DoH to the individual.

Research and development (R&D)

Research and development is an integral part of clinical governance. The 'R' (research) aspect is often associated with the generation of new, and testing of existing, knowledge. The 'D' aspect for (development) is often unsupported and undervalued in many healthcare organisations, e.g. within clinical governance, staff are expected to be research aware although little resource is allocated in supporting this need. One aspect of

Phase 1	February/March
Corporate objectives to executive directors	

Phase 2	April
Executive and general clinical managers agree objectives to address corporate objectives	

Phase 3	April
General and clinical managers and heads of department agree objectives of their respective departments	

Phase 4	April
Employees and heads of department agree individual objectives; personal development plans agreed	

Fig. 3.6   A model to aid the facilitation of CPD into healthcare organisations.

research development is concerned with establishing ways of enhancing health by the introduction of research. For more information on R&D view the DoH Research and Development website:http://www.doh.gov.uk/research

To promote evidence based practice a system for accessing, implementing, monitoring, supporting, supervising and disseminating research findings should be established to ensure that clinical practices and patient care are based on the most recent and best available scientific evidence, commonly referred to as evidence based practice. So what is evidence based practice? The following sections are based on McSherry and Haddock (1999) with kind permission of Mark Allen Publishers Ltd.

Evidence based healthcare

Evidence based practice is 'the process of systematically finding and using contemporaneous research findings as the basis for clinical decision-making' (Long & Harrison 1996) and is an integral part of the clinical governance framework, as illustrated in Figs 3.3 and 3.5. For the successful implementation of clinical governance for organisations and individuals, it is essential that all systems, processes, infrastructures and health professionals are developed using the principles of evidence based practice. To facilitate the development of evidence based practice the following processes need to be applied (Cullum *et al.* 1998; Kitson 1997; Swage 1998):

- Identify areas in practice from which clear clinical questions can be formulated.
- Identify the best-related evidence from available literature.
- Critically appraise the evidence for validity and clinical usefulness.
- Implement and incorporate relevant findings into practice.
- Subsequently measure performance against expected outcomes or against peers.

For example, to develop an evidenced based organisational strategy for clinical risk management, in ensuring the systematic delivery of appropriate and safe healthcare by the organisation and all its employees, health care professionals require regular clinical exposure and experience (Cullum *et al.* 1998) This is essential in order for them to become familiar and competent in rationalising the risks and benefits of a particular treatment, intervention or delivery of care, to deal with the patient's unique individual set of circumstances. It should only be allowed to occur following a structured period of education and supervision, and when the individual feels competent to do the procedure without assistance.

The continued clinical exposure, observations and experience of new treatments or interventions should in addition be supported by the relevant research evidence where patient participation is reflected in the final choice of treatment, intervention or application of care. The development of healthcare professionals to equip themselves with the critical appraisal skills required to rationalise the risks and benefits of care, and indeed to critique research evidence, requires organisational leadership and service support, sufficient resources and indeed a change in the culture to enable staff to work in this way. Therefore in order for evidence based practice to function within the context of clinical governance and to truly exist and operate effectively, the key components and structures illustrated in Fig. 3.3 are required.

Figure 3.3 illustrates that it is essential that efficient and effective channels of communication and information-giving are established to promote a culture that proactively develops infrastructures that nurture professional and practice development in the pursuit of clinical excellence. This can only be achieved by ensuring that the services provided are staffed with appropriately skilled, knowledgeable and competent practitioners who are then actively supported to further develop, apply and evaluate the care or service provided, with the aim of improving the quality and standards of care and treatment delivered to patients. Following the creation of an appropriate environment and culture which supports the development of evidence based care, it is essential to know how and where to access information.

Locating the evidence

The following is a guide to where research evidence may be obtained in supporting clinical practices:

- Libraries, local/national
- Voluntary and support organisations
- Clinical audit departments
- Centres for research and development
- Practice development centres
- Centre for reviews and dissemination (York)
- Professional bodies
- Local universities
- Information technology centres
- Electric computerised databases (CINHAL, MEDLINE)
- The Cochrane Library
- Expert advice

A fundamental problem facing some health care professionals after obtaining the relevant information or research evidence is the process of critical appraisal, i.e. how do you evaluate the information? Is it useful, reliable and relevant? This was highlighted by Swage (1998): 'many nurses (indeed all health professionals) stumble at the first hurdle because they are not confident about understanding research and reviews'.

Evidence based care and the need for critical appraisal skills

Crombie (1996), Sackett *et al.* (1997) and Swage (1998) suggest that critical appraisal is about considering the relevance of a research question, evaluating the evidence collected to answer the question and assessing the effectiveness of the conclusion and the recommendation of the evidence. In a simple way it is about systematically reviewing and questioning the stages of the research process, i.e. title and abstract, introduction/literature review, methods, results, discussions and recommendations, and asking the following questions (adapted from Crombie 1996):

- Is the research of interest?
- Why was it done?
- How was it performed?
- Who was it done to?
- What did it show?
- What is the possible implication for your practice?
- What next: information only, uninteresting or support practice?

Having had the education and training to critically appraise research, in the hope of practising evidence based care, why is it that so many healthcare professionals continue to base practice around tradition or rituals despite research evidence showing the contrary? Perhaps this is because of some of the barriers to implementation.

Barriers to implementation of the evidence

An enormous amount of literature continues to flood the academic journals relating to all professional groups, suggesting that the theory-practice gap continues to widen (Bassett 1993; McSherry 1997; May *et al.* 1998). To instigate evidence based care at a clinical level, perhaps organisations and staff need to become familiar with these barriers and begin to develop realistic strategies to overcome them. Healthcare professionals need to challenge these barriers in the continued attempt to improve their quality and standards of clinical practices in light of rising patient expectations and recent government reforms (Chapter 1).

The barriers that continue to be faced by many are:

- Attitudes towards research
- Lack of confidence, understanding and the skills to critically appraise
- Insufficient time within work commitments
- Lack of support from peers, managers and other health professionals
- Lack of resources
- Resistance to change.

Despite attempts to implement research evidence to support practices, many staff continue to experience difficulty with ensuring that the care and treatment they provide is evaluated effectively. Barriers are explored in more detail in Chapter 6.

Evaluation of the evidence

It is important that, following the implementation of research findings on delivering care and treatments, we continue to evaluate the quality, standard and effectiveness of our intervention with regards to the patients' outcomes or benefits to the service or organisation. There are many ways in addition to peer review that this can be achieved:

- Clinical audit
- Comparing standards against national accreditation, e.g. Kings Fund Centre, Calman and Hine cancer specifications
- Using a performance management framework
- Benchmarking: the use of comparative performance, i.e. comparing standards and outcomes against similar organisations.

Summary

Should efficient and effective systems of continuous practice and professional development, research and development, clinical risk and clinical audit be established, the overall cultural emphasis shifts from a reactive nature – i.e. acting on complaints from an unfortunate incident or on areas of poor practice or performance resulting from either an individual or service failure – to a more proactive nature, in trying to avoid the incident from happening in the first place (McSherry & Haddock 1999).

In order to make continuous quality improvement in organisations, teams and individuals, quality information is needed.

Quality information

For healthcare professionals and organisations to deliver quality standards, effective communication and information-giving are essential. Communication is defined as 'the exchange of information for some purposes' (Cherry 1978). This broad definition of communication is pertinent when exploring clinical governance because it emphasises the enormous task in hand for all healthcare professionals in tailoring their services to the client group and clinical setting and in exchanging the relevant information with the patient, carers, the public and fellow professionals. Information-giving refers to the 'the knowledge acquired through experience or study' Collins (1985). To provide quality information health care professionals need to have the knowledge, understanding and effective communication skills to exchange and receive information with and from their patients, carers and colleagues. The Audit Commission (1992) acknowledged that healthcare organisations and processes are complex, reinforcing the need for effective communication with patients about the clinical and non-clinical aspects of care. The report stated that 'lack of information and problems in communicating with health professionals usually come at the top of patients' concerns' (Audit Commission 1992). To address the concerns of patients and indeed the public with regard to poor communication and information-giving, many government initiatives were introduced to improve communications within the NHS (Box 3.3).

When referring to Box 3.3 and reflecting upon these documents it is easy to see the importance the government is placing on communication and information-giving to address the issues around poor communication and the stress and anxiety this causes patients and professionals alike. Effective communications are an integral aspect of clinical governance; furthermore communication within and between the key processes is vital in ensuring quality services. Communication and information-giving can

---

Box 3.3 Government initiatives aimed at improving communication and information giving

- *The Patients Charter: Raising the Standards* (DoH 1992a)
- *The Citizens Charter* (DoH 1992b)
- *Code of Openness in the NHS* (DoH 1997b)
- Data Protection Act 1998
- *Health Service Circular 1999/053 For The Record: Managing Records in NHS Trust and Health Authorities* (NHS Executive 1999c)
- *Information for Health* (NHS Executive 2000a)
- *The Caldicott Report* (NHS Executive 2000b)

---

be enhanced by auditing communications processes along with paying attention to the quality of information provided. In the *Code of Openness in the NHS* (DoH 1997b) the principles of good communication and information-giving are provided based around access to information, explanations, reasons for decisions and actions and information about what information is available. We believe that information should be given as outlined in Box 3.4.

Box 3.4 Principles of effective information giving

The information must be:

- Accurate
- Timely
- Current
- Easily accessible
- Clear and concise
- Audience specific
- Relevant

Note: When producing patient information leaflets or when sending information to patients, the Plain English Society could be contacted or any other relevant organisations such as the Charter Mark.

It is evident from Boxes 3.3 and 3.4 and the previous paragraphs that communication and information are important aspects in ensuring clinical excellence for patients, as well as being essential factors for the successful implementation, monitoring and evaluation of clinical governance systems and processes. The latter is highlighted when exploring the information required to demonstrate the effectiveness of clinical governance arrangements within healthcare organisations.

Information requirements for effective clinical governance systems

Quality information within the clinical governance framework is essential and information needs to be considered at three levels within the NHS: healthcare organisations, teams and individuals.

Healthcare organisations

As clinical governance is about sustained improvement in the care provided by the health service there is a requirement to demonstrate that this is happening. To do this a vast amount of clinical and non-clinical information is required. The Commission for Health Improvement (Chi) has the responsibility for reviewing the clinical governance arrangements of NHS Trusts, Health Authorities, and Primary Care Trusts (PCTs) in the future. Chi plan to perform clinical governance reviews (CGR) on a four yearly cycle, i.e. to review clinical governance in all NHS organisations every four years. An important aspect of Chi's CGR is the analysis of information provided by the organisation.

Chi have recently completed three pilot reviews of NHS Trusts (Chesterfield, Southampton and Sunderland), and have published their reports which can be found on the Chi website: www.chi.nhs.uk. In November 2000 Chi published a document *Clinical Governance Review at Trusts: Pre-visit request for information* outlining the information they require prior to carrying out a CGR (Box 3.5). It is evident from the three pilot reviews of NHS Trusts that some organisations have not been able to provide all of this information.

Chi summarise all the pre-visit information to help the review team familiarise themselves with the Trust's clinical governance systems and processes (of which communication and information-giving is one), select clinical teams for the review and focus on any particular issues.

All Trusts need to be able to provide this information. The final part of the Chi CGR process is the formulation of an action plan in agreement with the local National Health Service Executive (NHSE) office to address any shortcomings identified as a result of the review. To meet the challenges posed by the introduction of clinical governance we suggest that clinical governance leads in Trusts read and reflect upon this Chi document and use it as a basis for the development of the Trust's information strategies and in supporting their clinical governance frameworks.

Information for clinical teams

To facilitate clinical governance at the clinical team level, all clinical teams need information on how well they are performing. The types of data and information required to support this process can be categorised into those

Box 3.5: Summary of Chi pre-visit information requirements

The document is in two parts:

Part I: Information for internal and external sources
There are eleven sections to this part of the document. Each section is divided into two parts. Part I describes the purpose of the information, i.e. what Chi want to know about the organisation. Part II details the exact requirements such as organisational structures and processes as outlined in Fig 3.5.

Part 1: Information for internal and external sources

1. Trust profile-organisational charts, annual report, latest service and financial framework (SaFF), minutes of the Trust board meetings for the previous 12 months
2. Clinical governance strategies
3. Organisation and responsibilities for clinical governance
4. Patient/client/carer experience and involvement – analysis of patient surveys
5. Risk management-systems for: complaints, claims, critical incidents, health and safety incidents, hospital acquired infection and pressure sores, etc.
6. Clinical audit – annual clinical audit report etc.
7. Research and effectiveness – Trust R&D strategy, lists and description of R&D activity
8. Information, information management and technology – IT&M strategy, list of performance indicators, reports of any benchmarking exercises, etc.
9. Staffing and staff management – Trust's human resources strategy, analysis of staff surveys, information on sickness absence and staff turnover, list of GMC inquiries into cases of professional misconduct since 1998, latest Investors in People report, etc.
10. Education, training and continuing personal and professional development – Trust's education and training strategy, reports from the ENB, number and percentage of staff who have had manual handling training in the last 12 months, etc.
11. Information from other external sources – Latest CNST report and associated action plan, most recent internal audit reports, report of controls assurance assessment, etc.

Part II Extract of data from the Trust's computerised patient administration system

Trusts are required to make available a subset of data of inpatients and day case patients held on their patient administration system (PAS). The data is the same information, contract minimum dataset (CMDS), that all Trusts regularly submit to the nation wide clearing system (NWCS).

associated with quantitative (numerical/statistical information) and qualitative (patient and staffing experience) or a combination of both, as with complaints reporting you need numbers and trends to detect patterns, and also the qualitative information about individual complaints. Likewise this could apply to infection control issues. Examples of quantitative and qualitative information are:

- *Activity*: Numbers of patients treated, e.g. Finished consultant episodes (FCEs), Average length of stay (LOS) etc.
- *Quality* Quality indicators (QI), incidence of infections, complaints, pressure sore prevalence rates
- *Outcome measures* Data pertaining to improved quality of life for the patient for mobility, pain, which is obtained from the use of validated measurement tools, e.g. SF36, Hospital Anxiety Depression Scale, Barthel Index etc.
- *Readmissions*: These could be unplanned, i.e. patients returning to ITU, CCU or discharged patients being re-admitted soon after discharge.
- *Clinical incidents*: Any untoward incident that can potentially affect the patient's outcome, e.g. drug errors, breakdowns in communication affecting patient care, inappropriate care, etc.
- *Health and safety incidents*: e.g. falls, accidents at work, factors affecting moving and handling for staff and patients, etc.
- *Benchmarking*: Comparative information between similar clinical and non-clinical teams regarding team performance in standards and quality of care, e.g. stroke sentinel audit, UK trauma and audit network, NHS benchmarking service etc.
- *Accreditation*: Verification of the standards and quality of care/interventions against set standards, e.g. Kings Fund accreditation website www.kingsfund.org.uk, Charter Marks website http://www.barony.co.uk/chartermark.htm

Individuals (healthcare professionals and patients)

Professionals
The clinical governance framework contains within it infrastructures that facilitate the continued professional development of individuals and can be aligned to contracts of employment, personnel policies and procedures that are all linked to the concept of lifelong learning. To support the integration of lifelong learning and the continued development of staff, supporting structures, such as the following, need to be in place to encourage this process:

- Organisational objectives
- Performance appraisal (as outlined previously in this chapter)

- Personal development plans (PDPs)
- Principles of honesty and openness
- Access to education and training
- Access to adequate and appropriate resources
- Management support, e.g. whistle blowing?
- Proactive rather than reactive approaches to untoward incidents or complaints.

Patients

The public needs to be assured that they will not only receive the best quality service and care but will be active partners directly involved with this provision. Where required, special groups or individuals will be involved in service evaluations and developments such as developing service for individuals with disability, e.g. deafness.

In summary, quality information is essential to achieve effective infrastructures for the implementation, monitoring and evaluation of the systems and processes associated with clinical governance. 'Good communication (information-giving and receiving) flow is fundamental to clinical governance and accountability' (O'Neill 2000, p. 816). Accountability is our final piece of the jigsaw in Fig 3.3, which will now be explored in more detail in relation to clinical governance.

Accountability

Figure 3.3 illustrates how clinical governance is everybody's business, with all clinical and non-clinical staff responsible for ensuring that they are actively involved with managing and minimising clinical risks. This can only be accomplished if they have the necessary knowledge, understanding and skills to perform their roles efficiently and effectively. Continuous quality improvement is at the heart of all practices which are regularly monitored with a view to improved performance based on a foundation of efficient and effective channels of communication and information-giving. In essence accountability can be defined as 'the requirement that each nurse (healthcare professional) is answerable and responsible for the outcome of his or her professional actions' (Pennels 1997).

Accountability within the context of clinical governance could be viewed on three levels: organisation, team and individual, all having the responsibility for implementing, monitoring and evaluating the key components of clinical governance within their role. For example, the Trust board's chief executive is accountable to parliament in ensuring compliance of best clinical practice which is founded on the principles of clinical governance. This can only be achieved and demonstrated by having robust systems of communication, risk management, performance management, quality improvement programmes and effective information systems. Likewise a team (ward/unit/department/GP surgery) needs to have similar systems to demonstrate the delivery of best practice.

It is clear from Fig 3.3 that if you base your practice on these key principles your accountability to the public, employer, patients and profession can only be enhanced along with the standard and quality of care offered. In light of the recent healthcare reforms and media interest in healthcare (Chapter 1), it is essential that you become familiar with what accountability truly means. 'Accountability is like pregnancy – you cannot be slightly pregnant and you cannot be slightly accountable' (Glover 1999). To be truly accountable and fit for practice we would suggest that you address the following questions:

- What are the contributing factors for change in individual and professional practice?
- What might be the consequences of not changing or developing professional practice?
- How can you ensure that your practice is evidence based?
- How do you know that your practice is efficient and effective.

You will then be equipped with the knowledge, understanding and skills to support your professional accountability. If you familiarise yourself with the issues contained within this chapter and adopt the principles of lifelong learning to address any subsequent gaps in your own knowledge and skills, you will be demonstrating your ability to justify clinical judgements relating to accountability, legal and professional issues and subsequent advances in your practice.

Conclusion

This chapter has outlined in detail the key components of clinical governance and their relationship to organisations, teams and individuals in the pursuit of clinical excellence. The challenges for many healthcare professionals are not in describing or explaining what clinical governance is, but in applying and working with this concept in their daily practice(s). Chapter 4 provides practical advice and guidance on how clinical governance could be implemented to support the organisation, teams and individuals.

Activity 3.1 Feedback: Key components of clinical governance

It is evident from the contents of this chapter that clinical governance is dependent on having an organisational culture that is open, honest and transparent in the way it deals with untoward incidents, complaints and accolades derived from internal or external sources, i.e. staff or public. To foster this type of culture a managerial style that proactively encourages staff development and continuous learning is fundamental if an organisation aims to achieve continuous quality improvements. Quality improvements are the overriding aim of clinical governance, which is dependent on having the correct systems and processes in place to assure quality for the organisation, teams and individuals. The following systems and processes need to operate efficiently, effectively and harmoniously if clinical governance is to be successful at all these levels of a healthcare organisation:

- Risk management
- Performance management
- Quality improvement programmes
- Information
- Accountability.

Activity 3.2 Feedback: Performance management

It is evident from the section on performance management that several factors may have a positive or negative impact on an individual's, team's or organisation's performance, such as the following:

- Management
- Culture
- Environment
- Effective communication.

Issues surrounding either the individual's, team's or organisation's 'performance' are associated with the above factors, which are primarily communicated via two sources: the public's perceived experiences of a healthcare provision and the organisational evidence such as untoward incidents, clinical complaints and quality outcomes.

KEY POINTS

- Clinical governance is about promoting and achieving continuous improvement within healthcare organisations.
- Clinical excellence is dependent on having a proactive management style and honest and open culture.

- Innovations and good practices are shared and lessons learnt from not so good practices.
- Clinical governance is dependent on the unification, integration and harmonisation of six key systems and processes contained within a healthcare organisation:
  - Risk management
  - Performance management
  - Quality improvement
  - Information
  - Accountability
  - Communication.

- Lifelong learning, continuous professional development and the integration of evidence into practice through robust research and development infrastructures, are of paramount importance in achieving quality improvements within the clinical governance frameworks.

RECOMMENDED READING

Baker, M. (1998) *Making Sense of the NHS White Papers*, 2nd edn. Radcliffe Medical Press, Oxford.

DoH (2000) *An organization with a memory*; Report of an expert group on learning from adverse incidents in the NHS chaired by the Chief Medical Officer. Department of Health, London.

Muir Gray, J. A. (1997) *Evidence-based Healthcare: How to Make Health Policy and Management Decisions*. Churchill Livingstone, London.

NHS Executive (1999) *Health Service Circular 1999/065 Clinical Governance: Quality in the new NHS*. DoH, London.

NHS Executive (1999) *Health Service Circular 1999/154 Continuing Professional Development: Quality in the New NHS*. DoH, London.

O'Neill, S. (2000) Clinical Governance in Action Part 4: Communication. *Professional Nurse*, **16** (1) 816–817.

Pearce, P. & McSherry, R. (2000) Development: Making it happen. *Health Care Risk Report*, **6** (10) 15–17.

RCN (2000) *Clinical Governance: how nurses can get involved*. Royal College of Nursing, London.

Sealey, C. (1999) Clinical Governance; An Information Guide for Occupational Therapists. *British Journal of Occupational Therapy*, **62** (6) 263–268.

Squire, S. & Cullen, R. (2001) Clinical Governance in Action Part 7: Effective Learning. *Professional Nurse*, **16** (4) 1014–1015.

Wilson, J. & Tingle, J. (eds) (1999) *Clinical Risk Modification: A Route To Clinical Governance*. Butterworth Heinemann, Oxford.

References

Audit Commission (1992) *What seems to be the matter? Communication between Hospitals and Patients*. Audit Commission, London.

Baker, M. (1998) *Making Sense of the NHS White Papers*, 2nd Edn. Radcliffe Medical Press, Oxford.

Bassett, C. C. (1993) Nurse teachers attitudes to research; a phenomenological study. *Journal of Advanced Nursing*, 19, 1–8.

Cherry, C. (1978) *On human communication* ... MIT Press, Cambridge.

Collins, W. (1985) *The New Collins Concise Dictionary*. Guild Publishing Company, London.

Cullum, N., DiCenso, A. & Ciliska, D. (1998) Implementing evidence based nursing; Some misconceptions. *Evidence Based Medicine*, 1 (2) 38–40.

Crombie, I. K. (1996) *The Pocket Guide to Critical Appraisal*. BMJ Publishing Group, London.

DoH (1992a) *The Patient's Charter; Raising the Standards*. The Stationery Office, London.

DoH (1992b) *The Citizen's Charter*. The Stationery Office, London.

DoH (1994) *Corporate Governance in the NHS, Code of Conduct, Code of Accountability*. The Stationery Office, London.

DoH (1997a) *The New NHS Modern, Dependable*. Department of Health, London.

DoH (1997b) *Code of Openness in The NHS*. The Stationery Office, London.

DoH (1998) *Quality in the New NHS*. Department of Health, London.

DoH (2000) *An organisation with a memory; Report of an expert group on learning from adverse incidents in the NHS chaired by the Chief Medical Officer*. Department of Health, London.

DoH (2001) *Building a Safer NHS for patients: Implementing an Organisation with a Memory*. Department of Health, London.

Donaldson, L. J. & Muir Gray, J. A. (1998) Clinical Governance: a quality duty for health organizations. *Quality in Health Care*, 7 (suppl.) S37–44.

Donaldson, L. J. (2000) Clinical Governance; A mission to improve. *British Journal of Clinical Governance*, 5 (1) 6–7.

Edwards, J. & Packham, R. (1999) A model for the practical implementation of clinical governance. *Journal of Clinical Excellence*, 1 (1), 13–18.

Garland, G. (1998) Governance. *Nursing Management*, 5 (6) 28–31.

Glover, D. (1999) Accountability. *Nursing Times Monograph*. Emap Healthcare, London.

Kitson, A. (1997) Using evidence to demonstrate the values of nursing. *Nursing Standard*, 11 (28) 34–39.

Long, A. & Harrison, S. (1996) Evidence based decision making. *Health Service Journal*, 106, 11 January, 1–11.

Martin, V. (2000) How to manage, Part 6. Individual Performance. *Appraisal Nursing Times*, 96 (21) 41.

May, A., Alexander, C. & Mulhall, A. (1998) Research Utilization in Nursing: Barriers and opportunities. *Journal of Clinical Effectiveness*, 3 (2) 59–63.

Mayatt, V. L. (1995) *The CNST – How to meet the risk management standards and reduce financial losses.* HRRI Conference, Edinburgh, Paper Sedgwick UK Ltd.

McSherry, R. (1997) What do registered nurses and midwives feel and know about research. *Journal of Advanced Nursing,* **25,** 985–988.

McSherry, R. & Haddock, J. (1999) Evidence based health care: Its place within clinical goverance. *British Journal of Nursing,* **8** (2) 113–117.

NHS Executive (1999a) *Health Service Circular 1999/065 Clinical Governance: Quality in the new NHS.* DoH, London.

NHS Executive (1999b) *Health Services Circular 1999/154 Continuing Professional Development: Quality in the New NHS.* DoH, London.

NHS Executive (1999c) *Health Service Circular 1999/053 For The Record: Managing Records in NHS Trusts and Health Authorities.* Department of Health, London.

NHS Executive (2000a) *Information for Health.* Department of Health, London.

NHS Executive (2000b) *Health Service Circular 2000/Caldicott Report.* Department of Health, London.

O'Neill, S. (2000) Clinical Governance in Action Part 4: Communication. *Professional Nurse,* **16** (1), 816–817.

Pearce, P. & McSherry, R. (2000) Development: Making it happen. *Health Care Risk Report,* **6** (10) 15–17.

Pennels, C. (1997) Nursing and the law: clinical responsibility. *Professional Nurse,* **13** (3) 162–164.

RCN (2000) *Clinical Governance: how nurses can get involved.* Royal College of Nursing, London.

Sackett, L. D., Rosenburg, W. & Haynes, B. R. (1997) *Evidence based medicine; how to practise and teach EBM.* Churchill Livingstone, London.

Scally, G. & Donaldson, L. J. (1998) Clinical Governance and the drive for quality improvement in the new NHS in England. *BMJ,* 137, 61–65.

Swage, T. (1998) Clinical Care Takes Center Stage. *Nursing Times,* **94** (14) 40–41.

Walshe, K., Freeman, T., Latham, L., Wallace, P. & Spurgeon, P. (2000) *Clinical governance: from policy to practice.* Health Services Management Centre, University of Birmingham.

Williams, C. A. & Heins, R. M. (1976) *Risk Management and Insurance.* McGraw-Hill, New York.

Wilson, J. & Tingle, J. (eds) (1999) *Clinical Risk Modification: A Route to Clinical Governance.* Butterworth Heinemann, Oxford.

Chapter 4

Applying Clinical Governance in Daily Practice

Rob McSherry and Paddy Pearce

Introduction

Chapter 3 explored in detail the key components of clinical governance and the systems and processes necessary for its success. This chapter builds on the previous chapters by offering practical examples on how to facilitate the application of the clinical governance framework at an organisational, team and individual level. To make the introduction of clinical governance easier it is important that any organisation, team or individual is clear about what clinical governance is and why it is important to the promotion of clinical quality (Chapter 2).

Clinical governance is 'a framework through which NHS organisations are accountable for continuously improving the quality of their services and safeguarding high standards of care, by creating an environment in which clinical excellence in clinical care will flourish' (DoH 1997). It emerges from this definition that the successful development, implementation and evaluation of clinical governance frameworks are associated with 'two distinct elements – the mechanistic element of ensuring systems are in place, and the more philosophical element of producing a culture in which clinical quality can flourish' (Haslock 1999, p. 744).

To advance clinical governance within the NHS, all healthcare organisations need to establish their level of quality as required by the Department of Health in the Health Service Circular HSC 1999/065 (NHS Executive 1999). To achieve these standards within any healthcare organisation a baseline assessment of their existing organisational systems and processes is required. The baseline assessment is necessary to reveal strengths and weaknesses of existing systems and processes so that a robust action plan can be developed to facilitate the development, implementation and evaluation of clinical governance. The difficulty for many healthcare organisations, teams and individuals is, where does this process begin?

Introducing clinical governance into healthcare organisations

Given the importance that the government attaches to clinical governance, by making the healthcare organisations' chief executive accountable for the successful implementation of clinical governance structures in the pursuit of clinical excellence, it is easy to see why many of the leads for clinical governance are members of the executive board, i.e. Medical Directors or Directors of Nursing. The rationale for this is quite simple: clinical governance is about achieving clinical quality. Therefore it is important that any strategy is led by a clinician who has the respect and confidence of their peers along with an ability to influence and guide fellow clinicians through the change management process.

For all healthcare organisations the first step towards implementing clinical governance is the identification of clinicians to be given the lead responsibility for taking forward the development, implementation and evaluation of a clinical governance strategy. Having identified the lead person responsible for the strategic development of the clinical governance framework, clinical governance committees (CGCs) were developed as subcommittees of healthcare organisations' executive boards. The CGC comprised senior members of staff representing various professional, personnel and managerial aspects of the organisation, with an overview of and responsibility for maintaining key components of the clinical governance framework, i.e. clinical risk, quality, performance management and professional development, as illustrated in Fig. 4.1.

Figure 4.1 describes the hierarchical relationships between the management levels, professional groups and the key components of clinical governance. Each tier of the triangle is responsible for their own practice and accountable to the next tier, for example the clinical governance subcommittee is accountable and reports to the Trust board. Examples of how clinical governance has been introduced with various healthcare organisations are offered by Edwards and Packham (1999), Haslock (1999) and Starke and Boden (1999).

The CGC's initial task was to ensure that a baseline assessment of their organisation's capability and capacity to implement clinical governance was performed in accordance with the guidance issued with the HSC 1999/065.

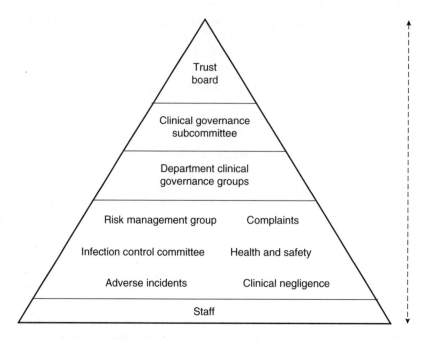

The dashed line illustrates how effective clinical governance is dependent on two-way channels of communication

Fig. 4.1   Management structure associated with clinical governance.

Clinical governance: what is a baseline assessment?

The HSC 1999/065 guidance notes provide in annex 2 a matrix of the standards requiring action by NHS Trusts, Health Authorities, Primary Care Groups and Primary Care Trusts. These standards needed to be agreed with the NHS Executive regional offices indicating how the key components of clinical governance were to be achieved for their respective organisations. A critical review of annex 2 reveals the main components of what a baseline assessment should consist of in demonstrating whether the organisation has the capability and capacity to deliver clinical governance. The annex can be summarised into four key areas as illustrated in Box 4.1.

The questions raised in Box 4.1 are synonymous with the information presented in Fig. 3.3 – the key components of clinical governance which describe in detail the systems and processes necessary for the successful development, implementation and evaluation of clinical governance. Figure 3.3 offers a framework that if used could provide organisations, teams and individuals with useful information regarding the initial clinical governance status and subsequent evaluations.

Box 4.1 Components of clinical governance baseline assessments

- Does your organisation have clear lines of accountability for the overall quality of clinical care and can this be demonstrated?
- Are there comprehensive systems for continuous quality improvement at all levels of the organisation?
- Is there a strategy for risk management and risk reductions?
- Does the organisation have an operational system for clinical performance management?

Table 4.1 offers a checklist for undertaking a baseline assessment of clinical governance based on the information obtained from HSC 1999/065 (Lim *et al.* 2000).

From the information obtained from the baseline assessment as shown in Table 4.1, an in-depth action plan should be formulated building upon the strengths and weaknesses identified by the baseline assessment in measuring progress in advancing clinical governance in the areas of 'performance, developing infrastructures, staff and board development, planning and prioritisation' (NHS Executive 1999, p. 2). Essentially the action plan developed from the baseline assessment should have realistic expectations in relation to:

- Aims and objectives
- Goals
- Actions
- Time-scales.

These expectations should be shared with all levels of staff. Having shared this information with staff, directorates, wards or departments, they need to conduct their own local baseline assessment and formulate an action plan to achieve their specific and overall actions identified by the organisational baseline assessment (RCN 1998). This approach nurtures the philosophy embedded in the concept of clinical governance by involving all staff from the outset in creating an environment in which clinical excellence can flourish. The application of this approach reaffirms the notion that the outcome of the baseline assessment is a true reflection and representation of the organisational, team and individual levels, making future strategies for change easier to manage because clinical governance is everybody's business – a view echoed in the following statement:

'If clinical governance becomes some sort of parallel universe detached from day to day management and practice, it is likely to produce a

Table 4.1 Baseline assessment checklist.

Standards	Full compliance	Partial compliance	Non-compliance	Additional comments
Risk management				
Risk management strategy and policies associated with clinical and non-clinical aspects of service		√		
Compliance with CNST standards	√			Level 2 CNST
Systems for reporting and detecting: equipment failure		√		
Managing performance Systems for reporting and detecting:				
• Complaints	√			
• Clinical incidents	√			
• Untoward incidents	√			
• Individual performance review	√			Consultant IPR introduced April 2001

Continued

Table 4.1   Continued.

Standards	Full compliance	Partial compliance	Non-compliance	Additional comments
Quality improvement				
Clinical audit	✓			
Compliance with NICE and NSFs guidelines/recommendations		✓		
Evidence based practice		✓		
Continuing professional development		✓		
Quality information				
Clinical information systems		✓		
Clinical outcomes data		✓		
Comparative data		✓		
Benchmarking			✓	
Accountability				
Policies and procedures	✓			All policies and procedures to be reviewed annually
Regular reporting to boards on efficiency and effectiveness of clinical governance		✓		Monthly reports to boards

resented bureaucracy that fails to deliver. It is only by embedding its principles and practice into everyday care delivery and organisation that it will succeed'

(Haslock 1999, p. 747).

To ensure that clinical governance does not become a bureaucratic 'nightmare' as alluded to by Haslock, staff must be fully informed of the managerial and strategic direction for the development, implementation and monitoring of clinical governance within the organisation, as outlined in Fig. 4.1. This could be done by having clinical governance briefing sessions and newsletters which ideally involve staff in the early stages of the process. Activity 4.1 will assist you in ascertaining whether your organisation is successful.

Activity 4.1: Clinical governance: baseline assessment questions

During the early stages of a clinical governance baseline assessment it is essential that healthcare staff can correctly answer the following questions to act as a starting point for the development of clinical governance:

Who leads clinical governance in your organisation?
Is there a manager responsible for clinical governance?
Who is the clinical governance lead for your directorate, team and department?
Is there a clinical governance lead for your professional group within your organisation?
Have you been involved with the baseline assessment at either organisational, team or individual level?
Have you had any awareness training on clinical governance and how it may affect you and what you do?

Feedback is provided at the end of the chapter.

Activity 4.1 is aimed at making you aware of how successfully your organisation's CGC communicated what and how clinical governance was to be implemented throughout your organisation. This stage in the process of developing clinical governance is essential in informing and involving staff before commencing the baseline assessment and subsequent development plan. Without staff's involvement in this process they are unlikely to understand and appreciate the importance of clinical governance at the clinical level; it will be seen to be owned purely by the senior management within the organisation. The clinical workforce may view this as yet another demand from government, construing it as not relevant to themselves or in the provision of services to patients. These misconceptions about clinical governance need to be tackled before and during the baseline assessment. Failure to follow this approach could be the reasons why clinical governance in some healthcare organisations is not owned and viewed positively by the clinical and non-clinical staff in everyday practice – a perception confirmed by the following comment

> 'much of the machinery of clinical governance at an NHS Trust level is now in place. However, it seems that clinical governance has yet to make a real difference at the clinical workface, and that changes in culture which it demands of healthcare organisations have not really begun to happen yet'.

> (Walshe *et al.* 2000 p. 3)

Following the development of a managerial and strategic framework for the development, implementation and monitoring of clinical governance, as illustrated in Fig. 4.1, and the informing of staff about this framework and subsequent implementation of the clinical governance baseline assessment, the next step is the writing and developing of the clinical governance action plan. The aim of the action plan is eloquently articulated by the RCN in suggesting that the:

> 'Development plan shows how your organisation intends to build on what is working well, how it plans to improve, what it is doing less well and how it aims to fill any gaps.'

> (RCN 2000, p. 7)

What does a clinical governance action plan look like and why are they necessary?

The clinical governance action plan should be developed in light of the findings of the baseline assessment undertaken by the CGC or nominated representatives. A format of how an action plan could be presented is offered by Garland (1998), RCN (1998) and Sealey (1999). The baseline assessment should highlight the strengths and weaknesses of the organisation in achieving the standards outlined in Fig. 4.2. The action plan should contain realistic targets directed towards improving infrastructures, performance and quality at organisational, team and individual levels. To some healthcare professions action plans are viewed negatively because they have predominantly been associated with poor performance and practices. In this instance clinical governance action plans should be viewed positively and used as a guide for continuous quality improvements and in the sharing of good practices and performances.

Clinical governance action plan

Appendix 4.1 provides a detailed template of a clinical governance development plan based on the five key components associated with the clinical governance framework as suggested by the HSC 1999/065 and McSherry & Haddock (1999). The template mirrors the baseline assessment offering realistic aims and objectives, and identifies lead personnel to take responsibility within given time-scales for achieving each specific objective. The difficulty for some organisations, teams and individuals is relating the principles of clinical governance to their own specific daily practices (Malbon *et al.* 1998). The remainder of this chapter will use case studies taken from the authors' own experiences to demonstrate how clinical governance can be applied to our daily practices at an organisational, team and individual level.

Box 4.2 For examples of case studies relating to how clinical governance can be applied to clinical practice read:

Kausar, S. A., Rowe, M. & Carr, J. (2000) Avoiding Medication Errors and Adverse Incident: the way forward. *Clinical Governance Bulletin*, **1** (2) 4–5.

Northcott, N. (1999) Clinical Governance No 1: Organizational Effectiveness–1. *Nursing Times Learning Curves*, **3**(2) 10.

Elcoat, C. (2000) Clinical Governance in action: Part 1 Key issues in Clinical Effectiveness. *Professional Nurse*, **15**(10) 622–623

Case study 1: Applying the principles of clinical governance to an organisation

A local hospital Trust has received a number of complaints from patients, and their carers, who have recently been admitted and discharged from the acute medical wards following a stroke (cerebral vascular accident). The complaints could be classified under the headings of poor quality care and poor communication.

Poor quality care
- Patients not having their privacy and hygiene needs attended to
- Development of hospital acquired pressure sores

- Failure to attend to nutritional needs
- Limited physiotherapy
- Delay in home assessment and discharge.

Poor communication
- Limited information about the patient's illness from medical staff
- Inconsistent information from the professional staff
- Failure to disclose information about patients' falls.

If each of these individual aspects of a complaint were reviewed in isolation it would be difficult to establish the severity of the problems associated with caring for stroke patients within this organisation. Having a clinical governance framework in operation within an organisation enables it to establish, understand and respond to clinical problems that are distressing to patients, carers and staff – a point echoed by Garside (1999):

> 'the big opportunity offered by clinical governance is the opportunity to change systems – to pull together different components and strands from the clinical and managerial worlds to improve things for patients.'

In light of this statement let us explore in detail how the systems and processes associated with clinical governance apply to the case study as illustrated in Fig. 4.2.

Figure 4.2 illustrates how the key components of clinical governance can be applied and demonstrated in action at organisation level. The case study demonstrates how clinical governance offers continuous quality improvement by working in collaboration with the various departments and their associated systems and processes (Northcott 1999).

In this instance when the complaints had been investigated the main issues were about poor quality not related to individual clinicians but to the systems and processes that clinicians had to work in. An analysis of the complaints revealed two areas within the clinical governance framework that required urgent attention: poor quality and poor communication, particularly information gathering and disseminating. The application of the clinical governance framework to this situation enabled a full review of the current standards of practices and this was subsequently reviewed against the best available evidence, and recommendations made and implemented in light of the findings.

The overall outcome of this case study reinforces the need for reviewing untoward incidents or failures that have a recurring theme or pattern at an organisational level based upon a systems and processes approach, rather than at an individual level. The outcome of the clinical audit based on the

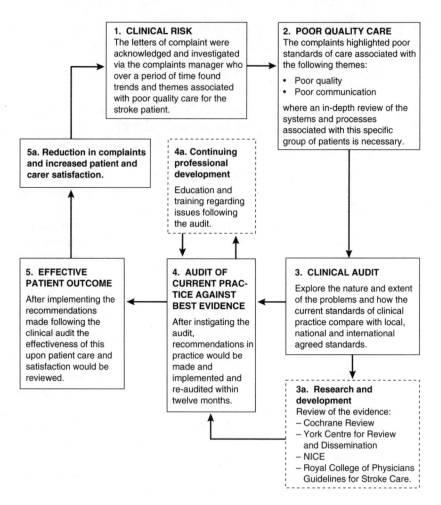

Fig. 4.2   Applying the principles of clinical governance at organisational level.

application of the best available evidence could make strong recommendations for the following:

- The need for a continuing professional development programme because the findings of the audit could have revealed a deficit in the clinical and management's knowledge with regard to best practices for stroke patients'/carers' care.
- The provision of a specialist stroke unit or designated rehabilitation area where patients receive high quality multidisciplinary care from specialist healthcare professions.

These points are more likely to be addressed as the recommendations are based on a thorough review of the current service provision using the clinical governance framework. A framework applied in this instance highlighted clinical risks, poor quality, and ineffective communications and information-giving which, if not attended to, could lead to increased levels of complaints and loss of local public confidence in this healthcare organisation. The long-term impact of this poor quality service could culminate in low staff morale and subsequent high levels of sickness and absence, thus exacerbating this clinical situation. As this statement describes: a poor lead organisation with a closed culture equals a clinical disaster waiting to happen. In this instance the notion of accountability becomes everyone's business.

The principles behind this case study could equally be applied to evaluating the existing practices for teams and departments in disseminating good or not so good clinical practices – a point reinforced by Smith (1998) when describing the effects of the Bristol case (see Chapter 1) where poor practices, performances and a closed culture culminated in higher than expected mortality rates for children undergoing cardiac surgery.

Case study 2: Applying the principles of clinical governance to a team

Case study 1 highlighted how the clinical governance framework can be applied to the organisation-wide situation in addressing poor practice and performance. Case study 2 explores how clinical governance can be used in a positive way to assist clinical teams to improve the services they provide.

An orthopaedic ward in a District General Hospital with a large elderly population had higher than expected incidence of fractured hips (fractured neck of femur). This demand on the emergency services led to increased waiting times for elective orthopaedic surgery such as total hip and knee replacements. The situation was further exacerbated by the shortage of qualified nursing staff within the orthopaedic specialty to care for this specific client group. In this instance no reported clinical complaints were recorded via the incident reporting systems or the complaints procedures. Clinical governance was used in a proactive way to support the healthcare professionals, managers and patients in developing new ways of improving the service and in responding to staff's concerns of not meeting government waiting list targets for elective surgery. Figure 4.3 illustrates the systems and processes associated with the application of a clinical governance framework to support a service development at team level.

Figure 4.3 shows how the clinical governance framework can be used to enhance the quality of a service at team level by the harmonising of the

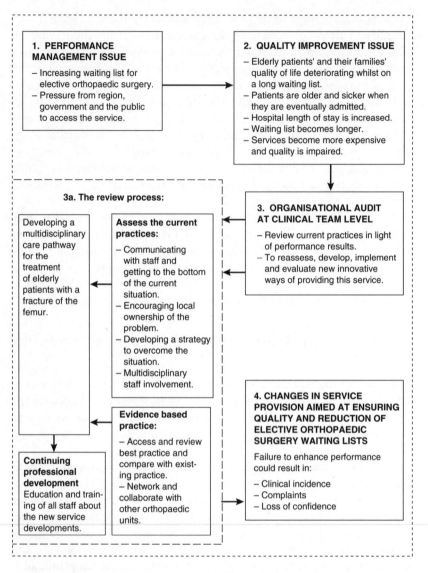

Fig. 4.3   Systems and processes associated with the application of a clinical governance framework at team level.

various key components associated with clinical governance. In this instance a *performance management issue* was detected via the feedback from regional offices, stating that the Trust's targets for elective ortho-paedic surgery were not being achieved. A *quality issue* was evident from several points of view:

- The quality of life of elderly patients and their families is deteriorating while the patients are on a long waiting list
- Patients are older and sicker when they are eventually admitted
- Hospital length of stay is increased
- Waiting list becomes longer
- Services become more expensive and quality is impaired.

In light of the above performance and quality issues an *organisational audit* of the orthopaedics multidisciplinary teams was conducted to see where improvements in the current service provisions could be made. The *review process* required all staff to be involved so that local ownership and participation in the development of the new services were agreed by all members of the multidisciplinary teams. This proactive collaborative approach to continuous quality improvement is vital for the success or failure of any change – a challenge that is perhaps difficult and sometimes viewed as being unrealistic in today's NHS (Northcott 1999). The review process requires staff involvement in both accessing and reviewing best practices in the development and application of the new methods employed in resolving this clinical situation. To resolve the issues identified within this case study an *integrated care pathway* was developed and introduced after communication, collaboration and education of all the staff in ensuring the most efficient, effective and reallocation of resources.

In this case study, 48 hours after surgical intervention the patients are nursed on an elderly rehabilitation ward with the appropriate staffing levels to assist with the rehabilitation process. An integrated care pathway was instigated in this instance to 'ensure multidisciplinary processes of patient focused care which specify key events, tests and assessments occurring in timely fashion to produce the best prescribed outcomes, within the resources and activities, for an appropriate episode of care' (CNST 1996). The integrated care pathway would ensure that an auditable trail of the patient's journey could be obtained and reviewed because 'the expected outcomes, frequently specified at different stages of the care pathway, are clearly described and any deviation or failure to achieve these outcomes or interim goals is quickly identified' (Benton 2000, p. 97). The drawback of this approach to providing care is that it can be viewed as cook-book healthcare.

The culmination of this approach ensures that the orthopaedic elective surgery is increased because the beds are utilised more effectively. Failure by the clinical team to address this issue in a proactive way with the support of management and the clinical and non-clinical staff could eventually lead to increased patients' complaints or untoward incidents, making the need for change a reactive one not proactive – an approach that would certainly have an impact on the healthcare professionals working within this specialty area.

Essentially case study 2 demonstrates how using a proactive approach to implementing clinical governance can bring about improvements for patients, staff and management by the use of multidisciplinary collaboration – partnerships in creating an environment and culture where all parties are involved from the outset.

As the saying goes, 'a problem shared is a problem halved'. How can we afford not to adopt this type of approach to promote continuous quality improvement?

The final case study in highlighting how clinical governance can be applied to the clinical situation focuses on its relevance to the individual healthcare professional.

Case study 3: Systems and processes associated with the application of a clinical governance framework at individual level

Case study 3 is adapted from the second case study in an article by McSherry (1999) in *Health Care Risk Report*, that explored the value of practice and professional development in assisting an organisation and individual to use the principles of clinical governance in daily practice.

A 38-year-old woman complains to her local hospital on discharge. Following her admission on to the acute medical ward for treatment of painful joints, she says a senior healthcare professional (could be a nurse, doctor or any healthcare professional who undertakes adjustments to extend or expand their roles) was abrupt and insensitive when inserting a cannula into her right hand. This caused unnecessary bruising and discomfort because they tried several times to insert the cannula without success. The woman stated that it was not until a more experienced member of staff saw what was happening and took over this duty from the staff member that the cannula was inserted on the first attempt.

Let us explore in detail how clinical governance may assist in overcoming this clinical incident associated with an individual's practice. In recent years a nurse manager, on receiving this complaint, might have rushed into establishing how this had occurred and who was responsible for such an incident so that disciplinary procedures could be instigated. This reactionary approach to management does not bode well in the context of clinical governance that promotes a blame free culture by the use of a proactive management style, as outlined in Chapter 3. Figure 4.4 illustrates how the key components of clinical governance can be applied to encourage the individual, team and organisation to learn and develop from this clinical incident.

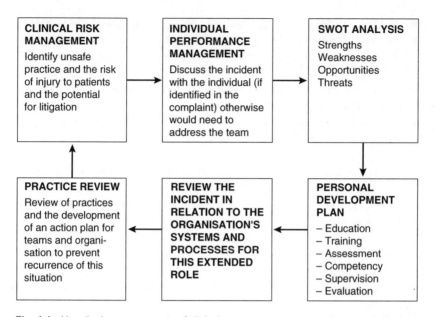

Fig. 4.4 How the key components of clinical governance can be applied to an individual.

In this case study the incident was reported via the clinical incident reporting system and was passed to the respective clinical manager for this directorate/ward to investigate and feedback the findings to the clinical risk management team for a response to be given to the client. To address and alleviate the situation the manager would discuss the incident with the individual and undertake a *SWOT analysis* of the individual's strengths, weaknesses, opportunities and threats. This would pay particular attention to the incident and ensure that the healthcare professional had the necessary knowledge, skills and competence to perform the role of venous cannulation. If it was established that he/she lacked the competency or capability then a personal development plan (PDP) would be jointly agreed and written. This would incorporate regular monthly evaluations with the line manager. The plan could cover education and training in cannulation, shadowing staff and encouraging professional development in clinical information and skills.

The period for the PDP would vary according to the individual's needs. The professional may have been unaware of the discomfort caused to the patient for many reasons – pressure of work, not enough knowledge or training, incompetence, etc. The development and implementation of a PDP could be seen as an important tool to promote quality and standards of patient care and of effective clinical risk management for the following reasons:

- A clinical incident was reported (patient complaint) and investigated
- An assessment of the individual's performance was undertaken (knowledge, skills and competency) against established research evidence
- A personal development plan was written, implemented and evaluated under supervision
- The overall outcome for patient and staff should be improved standards and quality of care.

An example of a personal development plan can be found in Appendix 4.2. In addition to supporting the individual to resolve the issues around poor practices and performance, a team or organisation could learn from this incident by reviewing their own practices and associated systems and processes aligned to the practising of intravenous cannulation. Case study 3 reinforces the concept of clinical governance at an individual level. It shows how practice and professional development can be enhanced under the key areas of clinical risk, performance management and quality improvement.

In summary, the case studies offer practical examples of how clinical governance can be applied to an organisation, team and individuals in the pursuit of clinical excellence. Case study 1 demonstrates how complaints about poor quality care can be a driver for continuous quality improvements at an organisational level. Complaints that are predominantly viewed negatively enabled a positive outcome to be achieved for the organisation by exploring and linking the key components of clinical governance. Case study 2 illustrates the determination of staff to improve their clinical services at a team level by collaborative working and partnerships, redesigning a new clinical service for the care of a specific group of patients and for healthcare professionals. This culminated in the development of an integrated care pathway for patients with a hip fracture, thus enabling more efficient and effective use of services and thereby improving the overall performance and management of the organisation. Case study 3 highlights how a proactive approach to the poor performance of an individual can be seen as a learning experience to themselves, clinical teams and the organisation.

Conclusion

In conclusion this chapter has outlined how healthcare organisations' capability and capacity to introduce clinical governance were initially assessed and developed by means of a baseline assessment and clinical governance development plans.

The difficulties for some organisations, teams and individuals is in transporting the findings of either the organisational or local development plans into clinical practice. To assist healthcare professionals to overcome this concern, three practice based case studies were presented and reviewed in relation to how clinical governance can be applied to these unique situations. The case studies systematically related how and where the key components of clinical governance could be linked to the various systems and processes of a healthcare organisation or Trust. Practical advice and guidance was offered throughout the case studies to enable the reader to apply the key components of clinical governance to the organisation, team and individual level.

Several themes emerge following the application of the clinical governance framework and the associated key components to case studies, which have the potential to inhibit or enhance the uptake of the goal of clinical governance – to promote continuous quality improvements and clinical excellence. Effective communication, collaboration and working in partnerships, and the development of a culture that values 'people' and their individual contribution to healthcare, are essential if clinical governance is to be realised in the modernisation agenda of the NHS.

Activity 4.1 Feedback: Clinical governance: baseline assessment questions

The initial stages of a baseline assessment should be concerned with ensuring that all staff can answer the questions in order to establish what is known and not known about the proposed systems and processes associated with clinical governance within the organisation.

If you are unable to answer these questions we suggest that you require education and training on how clinical governance is being developed within your own organisation.

KEY POINTS

- Individual healthcare professionals should familiarise themselves with their local clinical governance arrangements and infrastructures for delivering the clinical governance agenda for their respective organisation.
- All healthcare organisations should have a baseline assessment and clinical governance development plan to develop, monitor and evaluate the value of clinical governance to their own organisation.
- Clinical governance and its associated key components can be applied to three levels: the organisation, team and individuals.
- Clinical governance is everybody's business.

- A proactive management style and honest and open culture that values all staff, in seeking to learn from its mistakes in a blame free culture (where appropriate) is well on the road to successfully achieving the clinical governance agenda.

RECOMMENDED READING

Edwards, J. & Packham, R. (1999) A model for the practical implementation of clinical governance. *Journal of Clinical Excellence*, **1** (1) 13–18.

RCN (2000) *Clinical Governance: how nurses can get involved*. Royal College of Nursing, London.

Sealey, C. (1999) Clinical governance: an information guide for occupational therapists. *British Journal of Occupational Therapy*, **62** (6) 263–268.

References

Benton, D. C. (2000) Clinical effectiveness. In *Achieving Evidence based Practice: A Handbook For Practitioners* (eds) S. Hamer, & G. Collinson, Bailliere Tindall, London.

CNST (1996) *Risk Management Standards and Procedures; Manual of Guidance*. Clinical Negligence Scheme For Trusts, Bristol.

DoH (1997) *The New NHS Modern and Dependable*. Department of Health, London.

Edwards, J. & Packham, R. (1999) A model for the practical implementation of clinical governance. *Journal of Clinical Excellence*, **1** (1) 13–18.

Garland, G. (1998) Governance. *Nursing Management*, **5** (6) 28–31.

Garside, P. (1999) Book review. *Clinical Governance: Making it happen* (eds M. Lugon & J. Secker-Walker, RSM Press, London). *BMJ*, 318, 881.

Haslock, I. (1999) Introducing clinical governance in an acute trust. *Hospital Medicine*, **60** (10) 744–747.

Lim, J., Burton, T. & Bowens, A. (2000) *What Elements Should Be Covered In A Clinical Governance Development Plan?* Nuffield Institute for Health, University of Leeds & NHS Executive Northern & Yorkshire.

Malbon, G., Gillam, S. & Maysn, N. (1998) Onus points. *Health Services Journal*, 19, November 1998, 28–29.

McSherry, R. (1999) Practice and professional development. *Health Care Risk Report*, **6** (1) 21–22.

McSherry, R. & Haddock J. (1999) Evidence based health care: Its place within clinical governance. *British Journal of Nursing*, **8** (2) 113–117.

NHS Executive (1999) *Health Service Circular 1999/065 Clinical Governance: Quality in the New NHS*. DoH, London.

Northcott. N. (1999) Clinical Governance. Effective staff – 2. *Nursing Times*, 3 (4) 10.

RCN (1998) *Guidance For Nurses On Clinical Governance.* Royal College of Nursing, London.

RCN (2000) *Clinical Governance: how nurse can get involved.* Royal College of Nursing, London.

Sealey, C. (1999) Clinical governance: an information guide for occupational therapists. *British Journal of Occupational Therapy,* **62** (6) 263–268.

Smith, R. (1998) All changed, changed utterly; British medicine will be transformed by the Bristol Case. *BMJ,* **316,** 1917–1918.

Starke, D. & Boden, L. (1999) Case Study – how to make it work. *Health Care Risk Report,* **6** (1) 18–20.

Walshe, K., Freeman, T., Latham, L., Wallace, L. & Spurgeon, P. (2000) *Clinical Governance: from policy to practice.* University of Birmingham.

Appendix 4.1 An example of a clinical governance action plan

As discussed earlier in this chapter, the clinical governance committee would establish the strategic direction for reviewing the status of the Trust's capability and capacity to achieve the standards outlined in annex 2 of the Health Service Circular 1999/065. To comply with these standards a local baseline assessment was performed by nominated parties where a development plan was formulated outlining areas of good and not so good compliance. Following the formulation of the development plan the organisation should decide the best way to implement, monitor and evaluate the development plan. To do this successfully clinical directorates or departments need to develop clinical governance implementation groups or committees that are multidisciplinary, containing members from each of the main departments of the Trust, as well as key personnel such as clinical risk managers.

The clinical governance implementation group's responsibility is to oversee the development plan for their respective area by prioritising the work and producing a detailed project implementation plan for its completion. Below is an example of a written development plan that could support the organisation and directorate in achieving the standards outlined in HSC 1999/065.

To identify gaps in the present performance of the organisation and to bring these departments up to the desired standard

Aims

- To ensure all clinicians are involved in audit programmes.
- To ensure full participation in all four national confidential inquiries, e.g. confidential enquiry into perioperative deaths (CEPOD).
- To ensure that the clinical standards of the national service frameworks

(NSFs) and National Institute for Clinical Excellence (NICE) recommendations are implemented.
- To ensure that the clinical audit programme reflects the organisation's clinical governance agenda.

Objectives	Responsibility for actions	Time-scale: By
1. All departments to have a programme of multidisciplinary clinical audit which reflects the priorities of the Trust.		
2. All departments to hold regular multidisciplinary audit meetings to discuss the process of audit and the outcomes and to agree the implementation of change.		
3. The outcomes of these meetings to be reported to the clinical governance committee.		
4. Full participation in all four national confidential inquiries and feed back the results to the clinical governance committee		
5. The departmental clinical governance committees/ implementation groups will ensure that the clinical standards of the NSFs and the recommendations of NICE are implemented in all relevant departments, within the given time-scales.		
6. Clinical governance manager will coordinate the Trust's response to the visits of the Commission for Health Improvement.		

Risk management

Aim

- To assess clinical risk systematically and to introduce programmes to reduce risk.

Objectives	Responsibility for actions	Time-scale: By
1. The departmental clinical governance committee/group will:		
• Encourage individual departments to assess and prioritise their clinical risks.		
• Put in place systems to manage the identified clinical risks.		
• Further refine the clinical adverse incident reporting system.		
• Ensure the effective use of the clinical incident reporting system in all departments		
2. The audit department to regularly review the incidents reported with the Medical Director, in order to detect trends.		
3. The Medical Director will report to the clinical governance subcommittee.		
4. To coordinate clinical and corporate risk management, via the risk management group.		

Quality improvements

Aim

- To have in place a high level structure in the Trust to ensure that clinical governance is owned and developed at individual department level.

Objectives	Responsibility for actions	Time-scale: By
1. To ensure that all clinical staff understand how the Trust is addressing clinical governance and how clinical governance affects their department and themselves as individuals.		
2. To develop the work of the clinical governance subcommittee of the Trust board to ensure board level responsibility through the Medical Director/Director of Nursing.		
3. To further develop the multidisciplinary work of the departmental clinical governance committees/implementation groups.		
4. To continue to hold regular multidisciplinary seminars on the development of all aspects of clinical governance in the organisation		
5. To hold six monthly clinical governance awareness half-days for all departments.		
6. To continue the rolling programme of departmental presentations to the clinical governance subcommittee.		
7. To continue to produce the clinical governance newsletter on a quarterly basis.		

8. To produce an organisation clinical governance resource pack to be made available in electronic and paper versions to all personnel.		
9. To produce an annual clinical governance report.		

Continuing professional development

Aim

- To have in place programmes to meet the development needs of individual health professionals and the service needs of the organisation.

Objectives	Responsibility for actions	Time-scale: By
1. To ensure that all clinical staff have professional development plans, that are aligned to Trust priorities.		
2. To have in place a comprehensive system of appraisal for all clinical staff.		
3. To ensure that all clinicians achieve the accreditation standards for their respective professional body.		

Use of evidence in clinical practice and creating an evaluative culture

Aim

- To promote a culture of evidence based practice and learning from high quality research.

Objectives	Responsibility for actions	Time-scale: By
1. The audit department, working through the multidisciplinary clinical effectiveness group, will ensure participation of all clinical staff in the audit programme for their individual departments		

2. To ensure, through the clinical effectiveness group, that current practice and future developments are evidence based.		
3. To further develop the evidence based health care facilitator (EBHCF) to promote the use of best quality evidence to underpin clinical practice		
4. Through the EBHCF to teach clinical staff how to access and evaluate research evidence.		
5. To further develop and roll out the hospital intranet to disseminate information including research based clinical policies and procedures.		
6. To strengthen links with the local universities to develop research programmes that relate to the clinical work of the Trust.		

Quality information

Aim

- To ensure that effective safeguards are in place.

Objectives	Responsibility for actions	Time-scale: By
1. To ensure that the recommendations of the Caldicott review are implemented by all staff under the supervision of the Caldicott Guardian.		

Obtaining patients' views

Aim

- To monitor patients' perceptions of the service provided, including learning from both praise and complaint.

Objectives	Responsibility for actions	Time-scale: By
1. To strengthen the methods for receiving feedback from patients.		
2. To continue to publish these views within the Trust.		
3. To ensure that the Trust's complaints procedure is effective and that information is fed back to departments and individuals to ensure that the appropriate lessons are learnt.		
4. To consult with patient groups when new services are developed.		

Note: This is a guide to how a clinical governance development plan may be presented and should be modified to suit your own individual, organisational or local requirements.

Appendix 4.2 An example of a personal development plan

CONFIDENTIAL

HOSPITAL . . . .

DIRECTORATE . . . .

Name:

Position:

PERSONAL AND PROFESSIONAL DEVELOPMENT PLAN

Date: From . . . .   To . . . .

Preceptor/supervisor . . . .

In order to achieve the compliance expected/required of a healthcare professional undertaking the role of venous cannulation within this organisation, the line manager (name) . . . . and staff member (name) . . . . performed a SWOT analysis of his current position on Date . . . . Time . . . .

Strengths	Weaknesses
• Confident • Competent • Time management • Enthusiastic • Committed • Adaptable to change • Relevant experience in taking charge of the ward	• Inexperience with cannulation • Had no formal education or training with regards to venous cannulation (see one do one)
Opportunity	**Threats**
• Access to personal development plan • Support and commitment to develop the role of venous cannulation • Support	• Clinical time versus personal time • Lack of time to attend courses on cannulation • Time on the ward • Perception of colleagues in light of the incident

Following the SWOT analysis, a personal and professional development programme was agreed. The agreement is as follows:

- to hold monthly reviews
- to document after each session with regards to progress (see monthly review sheet)

- any new training/development requirements will be identified and added and dated as identified.

HOSPITAL . . . .

DIRECTORATE

WARD

Personal and professional development programme for

NAME . . . .   **POSITION** . . . .

The following development plan has been discussed and agreed by

Name: . . . .   **Date:** . . . .   **Signature:** . . . .   **Date:** . . . .
Preceptor

Name: . . . .   **Date:** . . . .   **Signature:** . . . .   **Date:** . . . .
Preceptee

Identified training and development needs to be met by agreed competencies	Training and development method	Time-scale	Evaluation of training
To develop knowledge, understanding and skills associated with venous cannulation	To attend the in-house educating and training programme for venous cannulation To shadow a senior experienced clinician during cannulation To practise cannulation under supervision of an accredited trainer To participate in cannulation audit within the clinical area		

Hospital . . . .

Directorate . . . .

Ward . . . .

Personal and professional development plan for NAME . . . .

Monthly review

Date	Progress	Signature

Chapter 5

Identifying and Exploring the Barriers to the Implementation of Clinical Governance

Rob McSherry and Paddy Pearce

Introduction

Chapter 4 offered practical examples on how the clinical governance framework can be applied to an organisation, team and individual in the pursuit of clinical excellence. For some healthcare organisations, teams and professionals the issues affecting the implementation of clinical governance are not associated with what it is and how the key components relate to practice, but in resolving barriers associated with the demands of a busy daily practice. This chapter explores the potential barriers affecting the implementation of clinical governance and how they can be resolved by focusing on models of change, teamwork, collaboration, partnerships, leadership and cultural issues.

The potential barriers affecting the implementation of clinical governance

Barriers are defined as 'an obstruction, a fence or wall, anything that holds apart or separates' (Collins 1987, p. 67).

Activity 5.1: Establishing the barriers to implementing clinical governance

Reflect upon Collins' (1987) definition of barriers and make a few notes regarding what you think the potential barriers are to implementing clinical governance in your area of work

Compare your notes to the themes in the Feedback box at the end of the chapter.

It would appear that Collins' (1987) definition of barriers is out of context when exploring the barriers to clinical governance within the NHS. The definition appertains to the presence of physical presence restricting movements. A critical review of this definition, however, shows quite the opposite.

Firstly, the word 'obstruction' refers to a blockage or anything that withholds or hinders the flow of something. If this term were linked to clinical governance, an obstruction would relate to anything that affects the quality of the vast array of systems and processes akin to its structures; for example, an obstruction in the channels of communication and information-giving between healthcare professionals and patients about preoperative risks and benefits associated with a certain procedure; or the failure to document an incident in the patient's healthcare records after a fall, where the patient/family complain about the incident asking for a full explanation several weeks after the event and no one can remember the event.

Secondly, a 'fence or wall' relates to boundaries, a term used frequently when exploring the relevance of clinical governance to the NHS. Boundaries can be used as a means of protection or a barrier to be climbed. Within the context of clinical governance, boundaries should be used to safeguard the quality of the services.

Thirdly, 'holds apart or separates' suggests the need for dividing or keeping something apart for a specific purpose, whether this be for positive or negative reason. Similarities emerge when relating this to clinical governance and the associated key components that are separate by name but not in function; for example, the need for clinical risks to be detected so that clinical quality is improved or maintained.

It is evident from Collins' (1987) definition that barriers can be positive and negative in nature, which is of immense importance when exploring these issues within the NHS and the context of clinical governance. For example, the clinical governance framework could be viewed positively at organisational level because it provides a means to improve quality by developing its systems and processes, but for an individual in daily practice it is viewed negatively because it is just another change without relevance to their daily practices.

The barriers associated with clinical governance

'It is important in the implementation process within a Trust (or other related healthcare organisations) that the requirements for and the process of clinical governance be viewed with enthusiasm rather than scepticism. It can really only be satisfactorily implemented on the basis of a welcomed initiative with the potential for developing real improvements in quality of patient care rather than a political imposition.'

(Edwards & Packham 1999, p. 13)

For some healthcare organisations, teams and individuals this is not the perceived norm. Clinical governance is yet another 'thing' imposed by government in response to the poor media view of the NHS because of the high profile cases that have highlighted inadequate standards and practices. Cases like the following:

- Bristol case – a consultant paediatric surgeon was found to have death rates for paediatric heart surgery significantly higher than the national average, and this only became known as a result of whistle-blowing (The Lancet 1998).
- Alderhay Childrens Hospital – a consultant pathologist at the Royal Liverpool Children's Hospital, Alderhay, Liverpool, removed the organs of over 2000 children without the consent of their parents. As a result of an inquiry he was banned from practising in the UK, and all NHS Acute Trusts had to perform a census of their pathology department and list retained organs. The Chief Medical Officer issued guidance on post-mortem examination (DoH 2001a).
- Shipman Enquiry – in 2001 a General Practitioner was convicted of the murder of 15 patients as a result of morphine poisoning (Ramsey 2001).
- Alitt Enquiry – a qualified enrolled nurse working in a paediatric unit was convicted of murdering four children and injuring nine others (MacDonald 1996).

These are all cases that have affected the public's confidence in the NHS, a confidence that requires rebuilding. Put bluntly, clinical governance 'is much more than a set of bureaucratic systems' (Harvey 1998, p. 8); it is a framework which is designed to help doctors, nurses, therapists and indeed all healthcare staff to improve organisational, team and individual standards and quality of care. To achieve the aims of clinical governance – reducing clinical risks, promoting continuous quality improvement and providing the best practices based on the best evidence delivered by professionals who have the correct knowledge, skills and competence via a system of lifelong learning – a shift in attitudes and culture is needed to a positive view of clinical governance rather than a negative one. Cullen *et al.* (2000) states that we need to change the culture of health care organisation and to do this 'we need to unlearn some old habits and develop some new habits'. This view is supported by Davies *et al.* (2000) who states that we will need to 'change the way things are done around here' to unlock the true potential of clinical governance.

The barriers affecting the implementing process of clinical governance are vast but not insurmountable, as outlined in Box 5.1

Box 5.1: The perceived barriers to implementing clinical governance

- Lack of understanding
- Fear
- No clear vision
- It's nothing new
- It's a passing fad
- Lack of time
- Lack of resources
- Tool of the management
- Lack of support
- Poor information/no information
- Poor leadership
- Ineffective communication

Note: This not an exhaustive list of the potential or perceived barriers to implementing clinical governance.

Box 5.1 shows that the barriers to implementing clinical governance originate from internal and external sources which can affect the organisation, teams and individuals, as illustrated in Fig. 5.1

The internal and external barriers affecting the implementation of clinical governance relating to the organisation or individual, as shown in Fig. 5.1, can be themed into several key areas as outlined in Fig. 5.2 and discussed here.

Culture

What do we mean by culture? Culture is defined as 'the skills and arts, etc. of a given people in a given period; civilisation ... improvements of the mind, manners, etc ... development by special training or care' (Collins 1987, p. 214).

During the late 1990s and early 2000s the word culture has become more prominent within the NHS, perhaps as a result of the many failures of healthcare systems, processes and the high profile professional misconduct cases, as previously mentioned. A common theme that has emerged following the inquiries of the recent clinical disasters and CHi investigations (North Lakeland Healthcare NHS Trust) is the use of the

Internal	External
Individual	**Individual**
• Lack of knowledge	• Lack of support, i.e. Peer, management or organisational
• Lack of understanding	
• Lack of confidence	• Lack of resources, i.e. personnel
• Lack of ownership	• Lack of time
• Fear of what's about to be or is being left behind	• Ineffective communication
	• Information
• Resistance to change	
• Ineffective communication	
• Information	
Organisation	**Organisation**
• Culture: openness, trust	• Political pressure
• Leadership styles	• Increased demand on already overstretched services
• Lack of ownership	
• Management styles:	• Increased performance targets
– proactive/reactive	• Public expectations
– change management	• Increased litigation
• Ineffective communication	• Lack of resourcing, i.e. financial backing
• Information	

Fig. 5.1 Internal and external factors influencing the implementation of clinical governance.

word 'culture' or phrases like 'open or closed culture'. The questions posed by some healthcare professionals are:

• Why is creating the right culture important to the NHS?
• How do you go about creating the right culture for an organisation, team or individuals?

The Department of Trade and Industry (DTI 1997) suggest that an effective organisation recognises that shared culture, shared learning, shared effort and shared information are the keys to high productivity and quality. For clinical governance to become a reality for any healthcare organisation, the cultural barriers outlined in Table 5.1 need addressing, as the rationale column suggests.

A healthcare organisation that is innovative, involving staff from all levels of the organisation and patients/carers, is an ideal foundation for the implementation of clinical governance – an approach advocated by Haslock (1999):

'for clinical governance to raise standards in a genuine and lasting fashion it must be developed in a supportive, blame-minimising, educational atmosphere'.

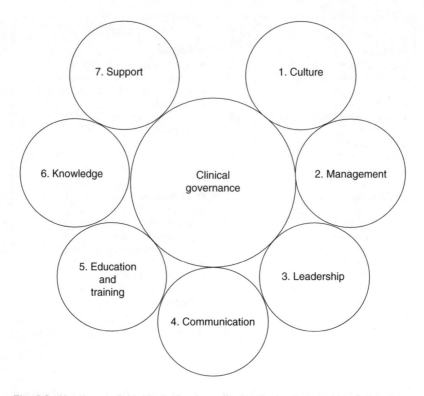

Fig. 5.2   Key themes linked to the barriers affecting the implementation of clinical governance.

The challenge for some healthcare organisations, teams and individuals is how to develop this culture within their respective workplace. The starting point for addressing the questions associated with culture is to establish the type of culture within your present organisation or team. Hawkins and Shohet (1989) identify five types of culture, as outlined in Table 5.2.

It is clear from Table 5.2 that a proactive culture of learning is the most suitable for the implementation of a system of clinical governance. This is because an environment or culture that seeks to apportion blame only leads to secrecy, mistrust and a failure to report mistakes, with a knee-jerk reaction to resolving the incidents; for example, a healthcare professional administers the wrong medication to a patient, which results in no harm to the patient. The immediate response of management was to discipline the member of staff, who received a written warning on their personal file – a classic case of reactive knee-jerk culture that actively seeks to apportion blame because of failure to adhere rigidly to policy and procedure. This

Table 5.1   Cultural barriers affecting the implementation of clinical governance.

Barriers	Rationale
• *Lack of openness*	• To encourage reporting of untoward incidents or practices. To state how you feel regarding a situation, whether it is good or not so good
• *Mistrust between employees and employers*	• To foster an environment where staff feel safe to whistle blow or voice concerns without retribution
• *Undervaluing staff*	• To create a feeling of confidence and pride in one's daily role and how that role relates to others, etc.
• *Not rewarding staff*	• Leads to low morale and inhibits the continuous quality improvements
• *Stifling innovation*	• Without nurturing continuous development the organisation and quality of care may not be developed and could deteriorate
• *Lack of transparency*	• Encouraging an openness where opinions within and external to the organisation are listened to

example demonstrates the element of culture that is bureaucratic, reactionary and closed, by blaming individuals.

Alternatively, in an open learning or proactive culture the incident would have been dealt with by exploring and establishing the facts before apportioning blame, with the systems and processes reviewed before any action was taken against the individual. This approach treats the whole incident as a learning opportunity for the individual and the organisation and where possible offers support, if needed, to the individual and patient concerned. The lessons learned from the incident are disseminated throughout the organisation, in an anonymous way to avoid naming, blaming and shaming of individuals, to avoid recurrence of this type of event.

It is evident from Table 5.2 and the subsequent example that for clinical governance to succeed, an environment is necessary that is open, honest, trusting and willing to learn from its mistakes and share good practices. The preferred culture to promote this type of environment is that of a 'constructive culture', a culture that:

Table 5.2 Types of culture (adapted from Hawkins and Shohet (1989) in Northcott (1999)).

Type	Key attribute	Preferred culture in achieving the modernisation of the NHS via clinical governance (the more asterisks the higher the preference)
Blame	A culture that seeks to address mistakes and apportions blame to individuals	*
Bureaucratic	An over-reliance on rules, regulations, procedures and policies at the jeopardy of individual personal judgement	* *
Mistrust (watch your back)	An over-competitive environment that seeks to embarrass departments and individuals and stifles developments	*
Reactive (knee-jerk)	Short-term management plans and dealing with the immediate problem. No long-term vision	*
Proactive (learning)	Encouraging learning and development. Learning from mistakes.	* * * * *

- Promotes learning
- Learns from experiences and mistakes
- Communicates to all
- Collaborates between all levels of the organisation
- Rewards, values and develops staff.

This type of open or transparent culture takes 'time, and requires working for collaborative results rather than relying upon domination or com-promise as a quick fix' (Northcott 1999, p. 10). Some organisations will require a cultural change to successfully implement clinical governance. This will not be easy and will require careful management and good leadership.

Management

The management style of a healthcare organisation will have a significant impact on how clinical governance is perceived and implemented. Management and leadership go hand in hand but there is a difference between the two. Marquis and Hutson (2000) suggest that management is about guiding and directing staff and resources and is concerned with having the power and legitimate authority for particular tasks and duties. Essentially management is primarily concerned with outcomes and the manipulation of resources to achieve the desired outcome(s). For example, in relation to clinical governance the chief executives of healthcare organisations are accountable to parliament for the implementation of the clinical governance framework, ensuring clinical quality along with meeting financial and performance targets – targets such as those outlined in the Patient's Charter (DoH 1992): to be seen in the outpatient department within half an hour of their specified waiting time; to be seen by a consultant within 13 weeks from the time of GP referral. These are all standards that require achievement through the process of delegation to other personnel within the organisation.

Management in this instance is about the transferring of roles and responsibilities to a specified team or individual for achieving the specific standards or desired aims and objectives. This collaborative and participative approach to management is the type that encourages a shared responsibility and ownership of what the organisation is trying to achieve. This is an essential attribute in the development, implementation and monitoring of clinical governance, where the success of the systems and processes as outlined in Chapters 3 and 4 is strongly associated with the specific management style of the lead for that part of the service. For example, if the manager or lead clinician is autocratic and not prepared to listen to the opinions of others, this will have a detrimental effect on advancing the quality improvement programme.

Previously in the NHS, effective management was valued more than good leadership. 'In difficult times, people need leadership as well as management' (Stewart 1996, p. 3) – an approach advocated within the NHS of today in addressing the factors that have led to the introduction of clinical governance and in developing new and creative ways of implementing the key systems and processes akin to clinical governance. In this instance management is crucial in both highlighting key leaders to take on the roles and responsibilities for advancing clinical governance and in empowering them to do this effectively without managerial interference. So what is the preferred management style for achieving clinical governance?

Management styles and clinical governance

Several theories have influenced the management of the NHS (Marquis & Hutson 2000). These can be categorised into three broad headings that have some degree of applicability to the implementation of clinical governance because of the nature of the management style used (see Table 5.3, adapted from Marquis and Hutson (2000)).

Table 5.3 Management styles and their applicability to clinical governance.

Theory	Description	Applicability to clinical governance
Scientific management	• Based on scientific principles • Efficient and effective use of resources • Having the appropriate staff and qualifications • Retaining and developing the staff • Valuing and rewarding staff • Cooperative relationships between managers and personnel	This management style is suited to the development of clinical governance because it links nicely to the notion of performance management. Performance management is associated with the continuous development and rewarding of staff
Management functions	• Planning • Commanding • Controlling • Coordinating • Organising • Staffing • Directing • Reporting	This type of management style is essentially related to the core aspects of the clinical governance framework because it fits in with almost all of the key components. For example, command and control are associated with 'accountability'. Staffing and reporting are associated with performance management and clinical risk. The planning and coordinating are related to quality improvement.

Continued

Table 5.3 Continued.

Theory	Description	Applicability to clinical governance
Human relationships management	• Involving staff • Valuing staff • Staff participation • Involved and shared decision-making	This management style pertains to the humanistic element of clinical governance and the notion of working in teams, sharing and learning from each when things go well or not so well, along with the involvement of the patients who are viewed as an essential asset when developing clinical governance.

It is evident from Table 5.3 that for clinical governance to be successfully implemented a combination of the three main management styles need to be applied at organisation and team levels. Each organisation or team should consider what their current management style is and what is the best way forward for them in managing clinical governance for the future.

The difficulty for some healthcare organisations and staff is not in eliciting what the preferred management style is or ought to be, but in overcoming the barriers associated with managing change effectively. For some healthcare professionals clinical governance is a new and alien concept that is associated with the reviewing of existing and the development of new systems and processes requiring change at all levels of the organisation. To this end the success of clinical governance will depend on how this change is managed. The following sections on change management and reaction to change are based on McSherry and Simmons (2001), with kind permission of Routledge, an imprint of Taylor & Francis Publishing Group.

Change management
Change is a complex process in which barriers are inherent, threatening the successful implementation of clinical governance. Utilising a change model can help guide the change process and help to reduce obstacles which may be encountered. Lewin (cited in Allen 1993) proposes a change model, the 'Force Field Theory', that has three fundamental stages – unfreezing, moving, refreezing – that could be useful when exploring the potential effects of introducing clinical governance within an organisation or team or for an individual.

Unfreezing.   For change to occur, individuals need to recognise that there is a need for change. Lewin suggests that for unfreezing to occur there is a need to understand the driving and restraining forces that exist. For example, a driving force may be the limited availability of information to support a change in practice and the restraining forces could be negative attitudes from the staff about this aspect of not informing them what is going on. This is a potentially huge barrier to clinical governance, where staff are expected to operate within the systems and processes but have not been informed about them or what their roles and responsibilities are within them. Whilst these forces remain in balance the situation will remain in the status quo. Unfreezing of a situation can occur when driving forces are increased and restraining forces decreased.

Moving.   This is where the organisation, team or individual begins to explore and examine the change or begins to accept or adjust to the changes being implemented. Teamwork needs to be nurtured and the emergence of key roles and responsibilities within the team highlighted. For clinical governance to work effectively staff need to be informed, and involved with the change processes. Management therefore have a duty and responsibility in ensuring these actions occur.

Refreezing.   Refreezing often occurs after a time, when the change has been accepted within the organisation or team and the individual staff settle back into a functional unit, where key roles and responsibilities are adopted, supported and communicated to and from each other.

Having decided upon the model of change to be used, it is essential to be aware of how individuals may react or respond to the plans to implement the clinical governance frameworks.

Reaction to change

Most healthcare professionals find change disruptive and by merely exposing the flaws of a particular practice or presenting research findings to support the rationale for change, you will still most likely face resistance. While individuals may resist, different people will respond differently. There are four main reasons why people resist change, as shown in Table 5.4.

The potential varied responses by individuals to a change are vast but should not be overlooked when implementing change on a scale as large as that required for the successful implementation of clinical governance. Managers should try and establish the views and opinions of the organisation, team and individuals about the levels of tolerance, misunderstanding and interest in clinical governance so that the barriers to

Table 5.4   Four main reasons for resisting change (adapted from Kotter and Schlesinger (1979) in McSherry *et al.* (2001)).

Type	Description
Parochial self interest	Where individuals may resist because they fear they may lose something they value as a result of the change.
Misunderstanding and lack of trust	Individuals often resist change because they do not understand its implications and perceive it might cost them more than they have to gain. This may occur where there is trust lacking between the person initiating the change and the workforce.
Different assessments	Individuals may assess the situation differently from those initiating the change and see more costs than benefits as a result, not only for themselves but for the organisation as a whole.
Low tolerance for change	Individuals may fear they will not be able to develop the new skills or behaviour needed after the change.

change can be avoided. The combination of effective management with leadership may help this process, as will be explored in the next section.

Leadership

Many people confuse management and leadership. Before we can proceed we need to understand the differences and relationships between leadership and management. This was eloquently described by Field Marshall Slim:

> 'There is a difference between leadership and management. Leadership is of the spirit, compounded of personality and vision; its practice is an art. Management is of the mind, a matter of accurate calculation . . . its practice is a science. Managers are necessary; leaders are essential.'

> (Slim 1996)

As mentioned in the previous section, managers are essential for the efficiency and effectiveness of an organisation and team. However, this is not to say that all good managers show the attributes that make successful leaders. For clinical governance to work we need leaders who can 'make others feel that what they are doing matters and hence make them feel good about their work (Stewart 1996, p. 4). This notion of empowering, involving and valuing staff is fundamental in developing the culture in which clinical governance will operate effectively. The essential attributes of an effective clinical leader are:

- Visionary
- Communicator
- Facilitator
- Advocator
- Critical thinker
- Doer
- Evaluator
- Respectable
- Knowledgeable
- Tactful.

A clinical leader will utilise these essential attributes to influence and develop the organisation, team and individuals by the execution of a specific leadership style which can be summarised into three main types, as illustrated in Table 5.5.

Table 5.5 describes how a democratic leadership style is potentially the most suited to implementing a clinical governance framework. The issue for some organisations, teams and individuals is in establishing their leadership traits and how to address them. Table 5.6 offers examples of personality types (based on Allen (1993) and Lancaster and Lancaster's (1982) adaptation of Rogers and Shoemaker's example of personality types, used in McSherry and Simmons (2001)), with their traits and applicability to clinical governance.

Table 5.6 shows that the innovators would come out top for supporting the implementation of clinical governance. However it is important to mention here that an organisation or team requires a combination and harmonisation of all of these personality types to achieve success. It would be impossible to develop a service if all involved were laggards or rejecters; likewise, if everyone were innovators who were never really challenged about their ideas or introductions of new systems and processes, this could result in advancing practices based on a minority opinion. The methods or changes advocated may not be the best way on this occasion. The way forward in exploring the issues associated with implementing clinical governance is about seeking the views and opinions of the staff. To ensure this occurs effectively, efficient channels of communication need to be operational.

Table 5.5 Leadership style and applicability to clinical governance (adapted from Marquis and Hutson (2000)).

Theory	Description	Applicability to clinical governance
Authoritarian	• Strong control • Gives commands • Communicates downwards only • Does not involve others in decision-making • Apportions blame	This type of leadership is destructive and inappropriate for the implementation of clinical governance. The whole style is at variance with the openness and sharing of clinical governance philosophy.
Democratic	• Less control • Directs by guidance • Two way process of communication up and down • Shared decision-making • Uses constructive criticism	This is the preferred leadership style for implementing clinical governance. It offers a strong vehicle for breaking down the barriers by the development of a collaborative, empowering and trusting culture based on a bedrock of communication and partnership
Laissez-faire	• Little control • Limited direction • Communicates well • Devolves decision-making • Group orientated • Does not criticise	This style, whilst containing some elements central to the development of a clinical governance culture, is not without its limitations. Constructive criticism is necessary with the clinical governance framework.

Communication

As previously mentioned in Chapter 3, 'communication seems to be about an interaction where two or more people send and receive messages, and in the process both present themselves and interpret the other' (McSherry 1999, p. 198). McSherry's quotation about communication relates to the need for a system of clinical governance because, 'without clear communication, it is impossible to give care effectively, make decisions with clients and families, protect clients from threats to well-being, coordinate

Table 5.6 Personality types and traits (adapted from McSherry and Simmons (2001)).

Personality type	Personality traits	Applicability to clinical governance (the more asterisks, the more applicable)
Innovators	Curious, enthusiastic and eager	* * * * *
Early adapters	Moderately enthusiastic, well-established group members, with high self-esteem. (Do not usually introduce radical/ controversial ideas)	* * * *
Early majority	Accept the innovation just before the majorities do.	* * *
Late majority	View the innovation with scepticism, do not actively resist.	* *
Laggards	Suspicious of change, discourage others by their negative attitude.	*
Rejecters	Openly reject change and encourage others to do so.	*

and manage client care, assist the client in rehabilitation, offer comfort, or teach' (Potter & Perry 1993, p. 24). Effective communication is an integral ingredient for the success or failure of clinical governance. It is of paramount importance in ensuring effective communications between and within:

- The various systems and processes associated with the key components akin to clinical governance
- Individual healthcare professionals both clinical and non-clinical
- Organisations such as Primary Care Trusts, Health Authorities, Acute Trusts
- National Institute of Clinical Excellence, Commission for Health Improvements

- National Health Service Executive, Department of Health
- Professional regulating bodies
- Non-statutory organisations
- Voluntary organisations.

A failure in communication between or within these organisations, teams or individuals could result in complaints about healthcare which are in the main linked to a failure in communications associated with 'staff attitudes, poor inter-team communication or lack of information for patients' (O'Neill 2000, p. 817). For the systems and processes associated with clinical governance to work in harmony, it is vital to have a culture that encourages open channels of communication between and within all levels of the organisation, teams and individuals. Failures to actively encourage honesty, openness and 'freedom of speech' contradict the philosophy behind clinical governance of promoting an environment where clinical excellence will flourish. 'Whistle blowing' and the reporting of poor practices, performance or competencies associated with the systems, processes or individuals should be encouraged via open two-way channels of communication between all levels of the organisation.

Communication can be enhanced and improved in the clinical environment by:

- Sharing of goals
- Information
- Learning
- Roles and responsibilities.

In this way a culture based on team work, partnerships and mutual collaboration becomes the norm. Clinical governance is not designed to work in a unidisciplinary manner; it needs teams and the individuals within the teams to collaborate, reliant on the efficiency and effectiveness of the communications processes.

Healthcare, and indeed clinical governance, is team-based relying on the 'direct or indirect support and influences of others, either from their own or other professions or work groups' (Northcott 1999).

This point is highlighted by the NHS Circular 1999/065 where multidisciplinary and multiagency collaboration is viewed as an essential component for improving the efficiency and effectiveness of the health service. Effective team working and multidisciplinary or multiagency approaches to care delivery are only truly effective where communication is continuous and seamless. For example, it would be fair to state that a patient's recovery from stroke is interdependent on multidisciplinary collaboration and effective communications, not individual practices. For clinical governance to function efficiently and effectively healthcare professions need to have the ability to coordinate patient/carers' care by passing information to and fro within the multidisciplinary team, a skill which requires effective management and leadership qualities.

If we find it difficult to communicate effectively with each other and with patients, what can one expect to find when it comes to reviewing standards and when faced with the challenge of implementing clinical governance into organisation, team or individual practices? For clinical governance to succeed it becomes evident that communication is of paramount importance as it is the unifying factor that crosses through all the key components. Communications should be based on the following principles:

- Appreciation and understanding of individual roles and responsibilities
- Open channels of communication between and within the organisation, teams and individuals.
- An ability to:
  - actively listen
  - express concerns
  - trust
  - work in teams
  - develop partnerships
  - collaborate
  - respond
  - act.

To achieve effective communications in supporting the implementation of the clinical governance framework the organisation, teams and individuals need to be adequately informed. The latter can only be achieved by offering the appropriate education and training.

Education and training

The education and training needs of healthcare professionals should be considered on a NHS-wide basis to inform and educate staff within all levels of the organisation about clinical governance. The education and training of all NHS personnel should be based on a 'need to know basis' where the appropriate information is provided about how clinical governance affects them and their role. To ensure that this happens, the employee and employer have a mutual responsibility to ensure that education and training are provided at a local level. The employee should make known through their individual personal development plans that they have a development need associated with clinical governance. The employer should seek to establish the educational needs of their employees, perhaps through the development and implementation of a staff 'clinical governance awareness questionnaire'. Likewise local universities providing healthcare courses need to develop clinical governance modules to educate both their pre and post registration healthcare students about clinical governance. The education and training programme(s) should be designed to best suit the target audience, as highlighted in Fig. 5.3.

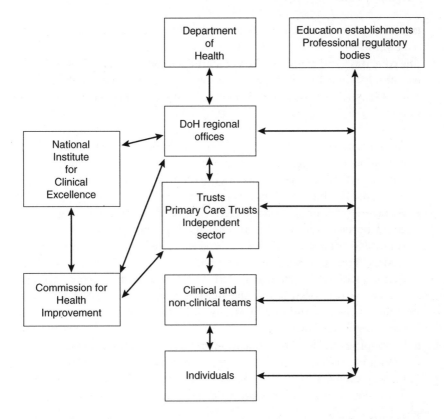

Fig. 5.3   The NHS structures that require clinical governance educational awareness sessions.

Figure 5.3 demonstrates the links between the various structures of the NHS and the need for education and training on clinical governance. It is imperative that all levels of the NHS are aware of their educational responsibilities in informing and educating their staff about the what, why and how of clinical governance.

The National Institute for Clinical Excellence (NICE) also have a responsibility to inform staff of the new guidelines to practice in keeping with the philosophy of clinical governance. Similarly, the Commission for Health Improvements (CHi) have a responsibility for reviewing the effectiveness of clinical governance arrangements for all NHS Trusts and health authorities, in the course of which the provision and effectiveness of education and training will be assessed. The most difficult aspect in the education and training of clinical governance, we believe, is in linking it to the organisation, teams and individuals and in releasing personnel from their daily clinical duties to attend clinical governance education courses, etc. (Phipps 2000).

Informing the organisation, team and individuals of clinical governance

The education and training needs of staff could be provided at three levels within a local healthcare organisation where the information about clinical governance is designed with a specific targeted audience in mind. For example:

- At an organisational level all new employees of the Trust would attend the induction programme where a brief presentation on clinical governance would be given, associated with an overview of the structures and processes linked to clinical governance.
- At a team/directorate level a specific education and training programme could be delivered via the 'rolling development programmes' where clinical governance is aligned to the specific activities of the team. Case studies, critical reflections and reviews of complaints are used as examples of where clinical governance fits in with practice, accompanied by networking and sharing good and not so good practices within the teams and organisations and where necessary externally to other organisations.
- At an individual level the education and training needs of the individual should be associated with learning needs established after the performance review, forming the basis of the personal development plan. These could be attendance on course, seminars or workshops.

The barrier for some organisations, teams and individuals is in establishing what they need to know – i.e. where clinical governance relates to them and their practices – and in accessing the information on clinical governance. This is where having a knowledge and understanding of clinical governance is essential if it is to become an integral part of healthcare professions' daily practice and not seen to be another obstacle to practice.

Knowledge

To ensure that all healthcare staff have sufficient knowledge and understanding of clinical governance the education and training should be targeted to specific audiences with relevant aims and objectives that relate to and reflect the realities of their clinical or non-clinical practice. All NHS employees should be made aware of the idea that for clinical governance to become a reality, it is everybody's business. To make certain that clinical governance becomes known and owned by all NHS staff, educational and training programmes need to be directed to the appropriate audiences. The educational programmes on clinical governance need to cover the key components such as risk management, performance management, quality improvement, quality information and accountability. Relevant examples and case studies are taken from real life situations to reinforce understanding and the relevance of clinical practice to their own practice.

The development of any educational programme for teams or individuals should be linked to demands of the local organisation or educational requirement highlighted via the educational confederations (previously known as educational consortia). Any devised educational programmes should be:

- Multiprofessional
- Collaborative in nature
- Practically focused
- Evidence based
- Utilising a variety of teaching and learning methods
- Competency based
- Evaluated regularly.

An education programme could be based on the example in Box 5.2.

Box 5.2 Example education programme

Aim: To provide an introduction to clinical governance.
Learning outcomes:

- To describe what is meant by clinical governance
- To describe the key processes and components of clinical governance
- To describe what clinical governance means in relation to individual practice
- To apply the concept of clinical governance to clinical case studies identified from practice
- To locate evidence and sources of information on clinical governance
- To evaluate the effectiveness of the course on the individual's understanding of clinical governance in relation to their practice.

All clinical governance educational programmes should be about learning from the practical experience gained in the workplace, with the learning shared and disseminated across multiprofessional boundaries.

This approach to shared and problem based learning is more likely to be successful, an approach advocated by the following statements:

'Learning in teams, developing multidisciplinary education and training across different agencies, is the way forward for creating learning environments. It will encourage healthcare professionals to work in partnerships in sharing ideas and solving problems that focus on what is important for patients.'

(Squire 2000, p. 1015)

'New approaches to undergraduate medical education, such as the introduction of problem based learning, joint education with other professional disciplines, should in time improve teamworking skills; the importance of team working has been emphasised by the General Medical Council.'

(Scally & Donaldson 1998, p. 65.)

To foster this new approach to shared learning and problem solving relating to the development, implementation and monitoring of clinical governance, healthcare organisations, teams and individuals need to be supported.

Support

The success of clinical governance will depend on the support and resources given within the various levels of the NHS to implement such a huge innovation. We believe that the support falls into two categories, internal and external, as highlighted in Fig. 5.4.

Figure 5.4 shows how the supporting infrastructures for the successful implementation of clinical governance depend on collaboration, part-nerships and adequate levels of resourcing at organisational, team and individual level. The support is not just about financial backing but the physical releasing of staff to develop their knowledge, understanding, skills and competence to deliver the clinical governance agenda at a local or individual level. Local support for staff could be in the form of:

- *Clinical supervision*: Offering a framework for staff to identify and explore issues about the quality of care delivered, along with the identification of education and training needs in enabling them to improve their clinical competence.
- *Reflective practice and critical incident analysis*: To help identify and resolve clinical concerns and share good practice.

Internal	External
Financial	**Locally**
• Funding for staff support and equipment, e.g. clinical audit, personnel etc. • Back fill costs for staff attending courses • The development of courses	• Collaboration with other healthcare agencies and patient/carers support groups • Developing partnerships with universities, education establishments
Resources	**Nationally**

• Education
• Supervision
• Time out
• Access to information
• Expert and practical advice
• Accommodation
• Equipment
• Support from management
• Trust board commitment
	• Links to the:
	  – Department of Health
	  – Chi
	  – NICE
	  – Professional regulatory bodies

Fig. 5.4   Internal and external factors supporting clinical governance.

- *Lifelong learning*: The need to ensure that staff have the support to continuously develop professionally.
- *Performance management review*: To offer support and advice in the organisation's drive for continuous quality improvement.
- *Clinical audit*: To support staff in the evaluation of care associated with set standards and guidelines.
- *Offering the opportunity for networking and collaboration*: To encourage staff to share and learn from each other.
- *Professional self-regulation*: Offering support and encouragement for the development of the professions' and individuals' performances as outlined by the National Clinical Assessment Authority.

National support comes in the form of:

- *National Institute for Clinical Excellence*: By setting clear national standards to provide clear guidance to the NHS on clinical and cost effectiveness across a wide range of health interventions, and the development of services.
- *National service frameworks*: Directed at raising national standards of care and reducing unacceptable variations in care provision, e.g. coronary heart disease, mental health.
- *Commission for Health Improvement*: To provide support by independently reviewing local efforts to improve the quality of

healthcare by the implementation of the clinical governance systems and processes.

DoH (2001b)

Without the correct and adequate local and national support for staff, to assist with their endeavours at an organisation, team and individual level to introduce clinical governance, the implementation of clinical governance will not happen. Perhaps this accounts for the government's section in the National Plan in 2000 about the 'NHS will support and value its staff' (DoH 2000, p. 4), directed towards resolving the fundamental barriers associated with the provision of support.

Activity 5.1 Feedback: Establishing the barriers to implementing clinical governance

The barriers associated with the implementation of clinical governance can be classified into seven themes:

- Culture
- Management
- Leadership
- Communication
- Education and training
- Knowledge
- Support.

By exploring these barriers, which tend to be viewed negatively, it is possible to develop positive strategies for the successful implementation of clinical governance systems and processes at an organisation, team and individual level.

Conclusion

This chapter shows how the implementation of clinical governance depends on resolving the potential barriers that exist within the organisation, teams and individuals – barriers which, if left unresolved, will make the linking of the systems and processes associated with the implementation of clinical governance difficult to achieve. These barriers can be classified into key themes associated with culture, management, leadership, communication, education and training, knowledge and support. As individual healthcare professionals, it is imperative that we understand the existence of these barriers and develop strategies to overcome them. Failure to embrace this challenge will make clinical governance difficult to implement in our daily practices.

KEY POINTS

The barriers to clinical governance:

- Refer to an obstruction or blockage in one or several of the complex systems and processes that make up clinical governance
- Can be classified as internal and external factors attributed to individuals or organisations
- Can be themed into seven key headings for which strategies require development in resolving their impact at an organisation, team and individual level: culture, management, leadership, communication, education and training, knowledge, and support

- Management, leadership styles and culture are three barriers which cannot be overlooked from either an organisation, team or individual level when considering the implementation of clinical governance
- A closer inspection of these barriers will offer positive and constructive ways of achieving clinical governance

- Adequate support is necessary
- Education and training for staff on clinical governance is essential.

RECOMMENDED READING

DoH (2001) *Assuring the Quality of Medical Practice: implementing Supporting doctors protecting patients*. DoH, London.

Stewart, R. (1996) *Leading In The NHS: A Practical Guide*, 2nd edn. Macmillan Business, London.

References

Allen (1993) Changing Theory in Nursing Practice. *Senior Nurse*, **13** (1) 43–4.

Collins, W. (1987) *Collins Universal English Dictionary*. Readers Union Ltd, Glasgow.

Cullen, R., Nichols, S. & Halligan, A. (2000) NHS support team Reviewing a service – discovering the unwritten rules. *British Journal of Clinical Governance*, 5 (4) 233–239.

Davies, H. T. O., Nutley, S. M. & Mannion, R. (2000) Organizational culture and quality of health care. *Quality in Health Care*, 9, 111–119.

DoH (1992) *The Patient's Charter: Raising the Standard*. Department of Health, London.

DoH (2000) National Plan. DoH, London.

DoH (2001a) *Interim Guidance on Post-Mortem Examinations.* 5 January. http:/
www.doh.gov.uk/postmortem.htm

DoH (2001b) *Assuring the Quality of Medical Practice: implementing Supporting
doctors protecting patients.* Department of Health, London.

DTI (1997) *Partnership with people.* Department of Trade and Industry, London.

Edwards, J. & Packham, R. (1999) A model for the practical implementation of
clinical governance. *Journal of Clinical Excellence,* **1** (1) 13–18.

Harvey, G. (1998) Improving patient care. *RCN Magazine,* Autumn, 8–9.

Haslock, I. (1999) Introducing clinical governance in an acute trust. *Hospital
Medicine,* **60** (10) 745–747.

Hawkins, S. & Shohet, R. (1989) Supervision in the helping professions. Open
University Press, Milton Keynes.

Kotter, J.P. & Schlesinger, L.A. (1979) Choosing strategies for change. *Harvard
Business Review,* **57** (2) 106–15.

Lancaster, J. & Lancaster, W. (1982) *The Nurse as the Change Agent.* Mosby, St
Louis.

The Lancet (1998) Editorial. First lessons from the 'Bristol case'. *The Lancet,* 351,
117, 1669.

MacDonald, A. (1996) Responding to the results of the Beverly Allitt inquiry.
Nursing Times, **92** (2) 23–25.

Marquis, B. L. & Hutson, C. J. (2000) *Leadership Roles and Management
Function in Nursing: Theory and Application,* 3rd edn. Lippincott, Philadel-
phia, USA.

McSherry, R. (1999) Supporting patients and their families. In *Caring for the
Seriously Ill Patient* (C. C. Bassett & L. Mahin). Arnold, London.

McSherry, R. & Simmons, M. (2001) The importance of research dissemination
and the barriers to implementation. In *Evidence-Informed Nursing: A Guide for
Clinical Nurses* (McSherry, R., Simmons, M. & Abbott, P.). Routledge, London.

McSherry, R., Simmons, M. & Abbott, P. (2001) *Evidence-Informed Nursing: A
Guide for Clinical Nurses.* Routledge, London.

Northcott, N. (1999) Organizational effectiveness. *Nursing Times Learning
Curve,* **3** (1) 10.

O'Neill, S. (2000) Clinical Governance in Action Part 4: Communication. *Professional Nurse,* **16** (1) 816–817.

Phipps, K. (2000) Nursing and clinical governance. *British Journal of Clinical
Governance,* **5** (2) 69–70.

Potter, A.P. & Perry G.A. (1993) *Foundations of Nursing: Concepts, Process and
Practice.* Mosby, London.

Ramsey, S. (2001) Audit exposes UK's worst serial killer. *The Lancet,* 357, 13
January, 123–124.

Scally, G. & Donaldson, L. J. (1998) Clinical governance and the drive for quality
improvement in the new NHS in England. *BMJ,* 317, 61–65.

Slim (1996) Cited in *Leading In The NHS: A Practical Guide,* 2nd edn (R.
Stewart). Macmillan Business, London.

Squire, S. (2000) Clinical governance in action: Part 7: Effective Learning. *Professional Nurse,* **16** (4) 1014–1015.

Stewart, R. (1996) *Leading In The NHS: A Practical Guide,* 2nd edn. Macmillan
Business, London.

Chapter 6

Clinical Governance and the Law

John Tingle

Introduction: defining terms

In focusing a legal discussion, lawyers are always keen to seek definitions of terms and to identify the parameters of discussion. Definitions and identification of parameters bring clarity and certainty. Clients can be advised where they stand and can organise their affairs accordingly. Can this lawyer's exercise be usefully attempted with the term clinical governance? Is there one absolute definition that everyone subscribes to without exception and are there identifiable parameters to the topic?

Reading this book, a number of definitions of the term do seem possible and the parameters of the topic do appear unclear. A lot can be seen to come under the term. In view of this fluidity of nature, it would seem appropriate to view clinical governance as one of those umbrella type terms, like accountability, patient empowerment or lifelong learning. With these terms the focus is less on the term or label itself, but more on the ideas behind them. When the ideas behind the label are looked at, commonalities can often be seen to emerge.

From the perspective of the individual healthcarer, clinical governance would seem essentially to be about doing your job well and helping to ensure the delivery of good quality healthcare and services. Legal topics relevant to clinical governance could therefore range from health and safety law, employment law, ethical issues and dilemmas in medicine and nursing law, to consent, negligence, complaints, patient rights, and so on. In fact the legal discussion could be almost endless because of the fluid nature of the concept and the wide range of topics that can be encompassed within the term.

In order to provide a reasoned legal treatment of relevant concepts the discussion in this chapter will be focused on the topics mentioned above.

Litigation in the NHS

It is clear that the concept of clinical governance is being applied at a very difficult time in the NHS's history. Litigation and complaints in the NHS have been increasing for a number of years and are now at record levels. The National Audit Office (NAO 2000) stated on the NHS accounts:

> '... reported liability for clinical negligence continues to increase within the NHS, with total potential liabilities of £2.4 billion disclosed in the accounts as at 31 March 1999.'

Written complaints received about hospital and community health services increased in the period 1999–2000 to 86 536. The number of written complaints received about general medical and dental services and Family Health Services administration increased by over 2% to 39 725, the third annual increase since the implementation of the reformed complaints procedure in April 1996 (DoH 2001a).

Almost every day stories appear in the press about medical mishaps with patients being injured, though there is little evidence as to why they occur (Alberti 2001). The notable medical scandals of Shipman, Alder Hay and Bristol have certainly focused the public's attention and have put the medical profession on the defensive. Add to these scandals the increase in health litigation and complaints, and we have a serious 'lack of confidence problem' in the NHS to contend with. The Government and the NHS do seem to be gaining back lost ground, however, with a number of patient focused initiatives such as the NHS Plan. This plan aims to put patients at the centre of the NHS and works from the clear premise that patients are the most important people in the health service (Tingle 2000). Some fundamental new organisational structures have been put into place to achieve this new patient centred NHS focus, for example the National Clinical Assessment Authority, and Patient Advocacy and Liaison Service (PALS). The Health Secretary Alan Milburn, set the scene for all this when he called for a new bond of trust between patients and the NHS (DoH 2001b) in a speech to patient groups at the Kings Fund, London on 29 January 2001. He stated:

> 'The NHS was conceived in an era of deference and hierarchy. The mantra that doctor knew best fitted the feel of the times. Those times have long since gone. But the NHS has lagged behind in its systems and in its culture, in the way it trains its staff and in the way it relates to its patients. We live in a different century ... It is too much a 1940s system operating in a twenty-first century world.'

He called for a patient revolution in the NHS.

Clinical governance plays a key part in the NHS Plan and is one mechanism to help refocus the NHS towards being patient centred. Clinical governance can also help reduce litigation and complaints in the NHS by addressing clinical competence issues.

Competent clinical practice is a basic and essential prerequisite for the effective delivery of clinical governance. As a matter of common sense, if you practise safely and reflectively the risks of adverse incidents will be reduced and quality clinical practices will be maintained.

How the courts determine competent clinical practice

A court could be called upon to determine whether a doctor or nurse has been negligent. The term malpractice is sometimes used (Stauch *et al.* 1998):

> 'Medical malpractice may be defined, broadly, as any unjustified act or failure to act upon the part of a doctor or other health care worker which results in harm to the patient.'

In order to succeed in a malpractice action, the claimant or plaintiff (these words mean the same thing) must show that a legal duty of care existed towards the patient, that the duty was broken and that legally recognised damage was caused. For the purposes of this discussion the focus will be on the breach of duty.

A patient may complain, for example, that pressure sores were allowed to develop and were then not treated properly. There was no initial pressure sore risk assessment done and the sores just got worse. The patient has been off work for a number of weeks and this, they argue, could have been prevented had the nurse systematically assessed them for pressure sores and then treated them properly. The nurse, the patient argues, is in breach of their legal duty of care by not systematically assessing them, and then failing to treat the sores that developed. The nurse has behaved improperly and malpractice has occurred.

The word properly is important here. What is meant by this term? Lawyers would not necessarily know what proper treatment would be; they are not doctors or nurses, though some could well be. They would ask for an expert report from a leading wound care specialist and ask them, not what they would have done, but what they would have expected the ordinary skilled nurse in the relevant specialty to have done in the cir-cumstances of the case. They need to determine the standard of care. The courts would not necessarily expect best practice but reasonable practice, though this is an issue of legal debate and conjecture. Legally, competent, proper clinical practice is reasonable practice determined by reference to the famous *Bolam* case.

Lord Browne-Wilkinson in *Bolitho* v. *City and Hackney HA* [1998] Lloyds Rep Med 26 at 31, said this on the standard of care and referred to *Bolam*:

> 'The *locus classicus* of the test for the standard of care required of a doctor or any other person professing some skill or competence is the direction to the jury given by McNair J in *Bolam* v. *Friern Hospital Management Committee* [1957] 1 WLR 583, 587:
>
> "I myself would prefer to put it this way, that he is not guilty of neg-ligence if he has acted in accordance with a practice accepted as proper by a responsible body of medical men skilled in that particular art ... Putting it the other way round, a man is not negligent, if he is acting in accordance with such a practice, merely because there is a body of opinion who would take a contrary view."'

Over the years the courts have been seen to be reluctant to challenge what experts have said about reasonable medical practices when assessing the standard of care, being unduly deferential to doctors, a theme made clear by Britain's most senior judge, the Lord Chief Justice, Lord Woolf (*The Times* 2001):

> '... until recently the courts treated the medical profession with exces-sive deference, but recently the position has changed ... The over deferential approach is captured by the phrase "Doctor knows best". The contemporary approach is a more critical approach. It could be said to be that Doctor knows best if he acts reasonably and logically and gets his facts right."'

The courts can be seen to have adopted a more proactive approach to testing medical evidence and determining the standard of care. The *Bolitho* case is the baseline case for the new approach.

The case involved a two-year-old plaintiff who was re-admitted to hospital on 16 January 1984 after suffering a serious bout of the croup. On 17 January his condition deteriorated and there were two occasions where he had episodes of acute breathing problems. Twice the nurse observing him summoned the paediatric registrar but there was no response to the calls. The plaintiff suffered a third episode, which led to cardiac arrest and severe anoxic brain damage. It was accepted for the defendant that the failure of doctors to attend amounted to a breach of the duty of care. However it was claimed that had they attended they would not have intubated.

> 'Although this was a defence based essentially on lack of causation ... to succeed it required the court to accept that the hypothetical failure to intubate in such a case would not itself have been a breach of duty. In this regard, the defendant adduced evidence from a number of expert witnesses to the effect that, faced with a patient exhibiting the plaintiff's history and symptoms, they too would not intubate ... The House of Lords agreed that the hypothetical decision not to intubate the plaintiff would have been in accord with responsible medical practice.'
>
> (Stauch *et al.* 1998)

The plaintiff lost his case. Lord Browne-Wilkinson stated the following:

> '... [I]n my view, the court is not bound to hold that a defendant doctor escapes liability for negligent treatment or diagnosis just because he leads evidence from a number of medical experts who are genuinely of opinion that the defendant's treatment or diagnosis accorded with sound medical practice ... The use of these adjectives responsible, reasonable and respectable all show that the court has to be satisfied that the exponents of the body of opinion relied upon can demonstrate that such opinion has a logical basis. In particular in cases involving, as they so often do, the weighing of risks against benefits, the judge before accepting a body of opinion as being responsible, reasonable, or respectable, will need to be satisfied that, in forming their views, the experts have directed their minds to the question of comparative risks and benefits and have reached a defensible conclusion on the matter'.
>
> (p. 33)

The *Bolitho* case reconsidered the *Bolam* test and placed it within context. *Bolam* has been returned to its proper limits and appropriate context, as Brazier and Miola (2000) conclude on the *Bolitho* decision:

> 'The decision does, however signal judicial will, at the highest level, to return *Bolam* to its proper context. Together with the many other factors prompting change, inappropriate deference to medical opinion should be replaced by legal principles which recognise the imperative to listen to both doctors and patients and which acknowledge that the medical professional is just as much required to justify his or her practice as the architect or solicitor.'

The court's contemporary approach to determining the standard of care in medical malpractice can be regarded as an evidence based approach, which fits in well with clinical governance. Foster (1998) feels that evidence based medicine might begin to play a part in malpractice litigation after the *Bolitho* case:

'If the published evidence makes a wholly one-sided case against a particular medical practice, it will be difficult for any expert to say that its adoption by the defendant was reasonable, even though he or she is in august medical company in doing so.'

The law and clinical guidelines

Judges today will now be more influenced by national and local clinical guidelines issued by hospitals, NICE, the Royal Medical Colleges and other bodies that produce guidelines. This can be seen in the case of *Penney, Palmer and Cannon* v. *East Kent Health Authority* [2000] Lloyds Rep Med 41, discussed by Tingle and Rodgers (1999). This case concerned cervical smear tests and negligence allegations concerning interpretation of findings. Some slides had been labelled negatively when they should not have been and there was no medical follow-up for the claimants who subsequently went on to develop invasive adenocarcinoma of the cervix and had to undergo surgery, which included a hysterectomy. The Court of Appeal held, dismissing the Health Authority's appeal, that because of the observable abnormalities on the slides they should not have been labelled negative. The standards of the CSP (cervical screening programme) were not complied with and consequently the Health Authority were liable in negligence. The trial judge had relied on a test of screener satisfaction known as 'the absolute confidence test', which according to the judge all the experts seemed to endorse. The trial judge had used this test in deciding the issue of the correct standard of care and whether this standard had been met. This test is incorporated into the clinical guidelines of the CSP.

This case shows clinical guidelines influencing judges and is a theme which should continue as NICE issues more guidelines.

The practice of evidence based healthcare based on clinical guidelines is one way of demonstrating effective clinical governance. The courts would seem to support and use this approach in assessing whether malpractice has taken place or not. It could well be argued that reasonable clinical practice is no longer the acceptable judicial benchmark of appropriateness of clinical conduct. If most healthcarers are practising evidence based best clinical practice, then surely the standard shifts from reasonable to best practice? In time cases will clarify this point.

Personal updating: knowledge and clinical guidelines

Professional staff development is an important aspect to demonstrating clinical governance and is the hallmark of a professional person. We would all expect professionals to keep up to date with changes and developments in their field of expertise. We rely on them and do not have the skill to second-guess them. In the health care context the expectations of professional updating are no different. It is possible that a malpractice case could be brought by a patient who argues that the doctor or nurse was negligent in not applying an appropriate clinical guideline which would have helped them make a full recovery, or even some widely available research. A case could proceed on the basis of negligence through ignorance. A court would take the view that the reasonable doctor or nurse would be expected to keep up with professional developments in their sphere of practice, but what does this really entail? A doctor or nurse may read one article in the professional press about treating one condition and another may come out the following week advocating a different course of treatment. It is often said that medicine is not a science but a scientific based art.

On the present state of the law, minority medical or nursing opinion can still be *Bolam* reasonable with the caveat that the court will test the views. The courts will look for a logical basis and a risk benefit analysis. Clinical guidelines, nationally endorsed, may assist the court but would not be determinative. Each case will often depend on its own facts. Clinical guidelines do not suspend clinical autonomy. There is often more than one reasonable and logical way to care for a patient. A patient's condition may also contra-indicate the application of the guideline or treatment. The healthcarer should always be prepared to advance a reasonable reason for not following the guideline or the usual course of treatment. Two cases assist on this issue.

In the case of *Crawford* v. *Board of Governors of Charing Cross Hospital* (*The Times* 8 December 1953) the plaintiff developed brachial palsy as a result of his arm being kept in an extended position, at an angle of 80° from the body position, during an operation. Six months before an article had appeared in the *Lancet* pointing out this danger. The anaesthetist had not read the article in question and the judge at first instance, Gerrard J, held the defendants liable for negligence. The Court of Appeal allowed the hospital's appeal and found the anaesthetist not negligent. Lord Denning stated that:

'it would, I think, be putting too high a burden on a medical man to say that he has to read every article appearing in the current medical press; and it would be quite wrong to suggest that a medical man is negligent because he does not at once put into operation the suggestions which some contributor or other might make in a medical journal. The time may come in a particular case when a new recommendation may be so well proved and so well known, and so well accepted that it should be adopted, but that was not so in this case.'

(Mason & McCall Smith 1999)

Mason and McCall Smith (1999) comment:

'Failure to read a single article, it was said, may be excusable, while disregard of a series of warnings in the medical press could well be evidence of negligence. In view of the rapid progress currently being made in many areas of medicine, and in view of the amount of information confronting the average doctor, it is unreasonable to expect a doctor to be aware of every development in his field. At the same time, he must be reasonably up to date and must know of major developments ... The practice of medicine has, however, become increasingly based on principles of scientific elucidation and report and the pressure on doctors to keep abreast of current developments is now considerable. It is no longer possible for a doctor to coast along on the basis of long experience; such an attitude has been firmly discredited not only in medicine but in many other professions and callings.'

The views expressed by the authors are the attitude that courts would take today. *Crawford* was a case in 1953; the information technology age is now firmly with us, though a number of hospitals in my experience have yet to firmly grasp the technology challenges and have not developed intranets which allow easy access to guideline databases.

A more contemporary case on staff updating is *Gascoine* v. *Ian Sheridan and Co and Latham* [1994] 5 Med LR 437. This case concerned a number of issues, one of which was the responsibility of a consultant to keep informed about changes and developments in his specialty. Mitchell J said that the consultant in the case was a very busy man 'who clearly had a responsibility to keep himself generally informed on mainstream changes in diagnosis treatment and practice through the mainstream literature such as the leading textbooks and *The Journal of Obstetrics and Gynaecology*'. The judge went on to say that it would be unreasonable for the consultant to 'acquaint himself with the content of the more obscure journals'.

A balance has to be drawn. The healthcarer should, at the very least, be prepared to demonstrate a systematic updating regime; just saying that you do not have the time to keep up to date is not enough. An awareness of the main clinical guidelines in the relevant specialty should also be demonstrated.

Good guidelines practice

We have seen that clinical guidelines can be used to convey evidence based practice. Effective evidence based practice demonstrates clinical governance in action.

It is always good common-sense practice to date and sign a clinical guideline, and say who was involved in drafting it and what evidence was used. Always build in review dates. If you do not, how can you say that best practice is being followed? Practice changes, so a guideline should be reviewed. It is also worth stating on the guideline that the user must always use their own clinical judgement and that the guideline does not suspend this. These are common-sense steps, as guidelines could conceivably become the subject of legal actions. A patient could argue that a guideline was negligently designed and they have suffered as a result, or that another guideline should have been used. We have seen in the *Penney* case above how courts can treat guidelines. The DoH also produces useful advice on using clinical guidelines (DoH 1996) and identifies a number of legal considerations:

'(1) the objectives for the clinical guidelines need to be clear, and clearly stated. This will affect their subsequent legal standing;
(2) the intended use and applicability of clinical guidelines should be spelt out clearly, in the introduction;
(3) the guidelines must make clear for whom they are intended. The recommendations will usually be intended for a particular group of practitioners;
(4) clinical guidelines that no longer reflect best practice might conceivably become actionable, and developers need to incorporate specific statements about their validity and review procedure;
(5) they should be constructed in such a way that allows deviation and does not suffocate initiative that might bring about further improvements;
(6) the development of clinical guidelines must involve all the relevant professions and managers.'

This booklet provides lots of common-sense advice and should be read in conjunction with the advice offered on the NICE website: www.nice.org.uk.

Guideline developers need to create in essence an audit trail of their work as the information will prove useful in defending any claim of malpractice.

In conclusion, the law can be seen as an important mechanism to advance clinical governance. The courts are sensitive to the issues of evidence based practice and the need to test clinical practice. Judges are not as deferential as they once were. Litigation and complaints are on the increase but the Government can be seen to be developing key strategies to instil more confidence in the NHS. Clinical governance is just one tool being used and there are a number of others. The patient is to be viewed as king in the new NHS.

Professionals have a legal duty to keep up to date and cases have gone to court on this area. Clinical guidelines are an important quality development tool and a way of demonstrating the existence of the practice of evidence based care and the operation of clinical governance. The courts remain the final arbiters of what is acceptable clinical practice and they are the ultimate and final mechanism of clinical accountability.

References

Alberti, K. G. M. M. (2001) Medical errors: a common problem. *BMJ*, 322, 3 March, 501.

Brazier, M. & Miola, J (2000) Bye–bye Bolam: a medical litigation revolution? *Medical Law Review*, 8 (1) Spring, 85–114.

DoH (1996) *Clinical Guidelines, Using Clinical Guidelines to Improve Patient Care within the NHS*. Department of Health, London.

DoH (2001a) *Statistical Press Notice, Handling complaints: monitoring the NHS complaints procedure, England, 1999–00*. Department of Health Press Release, 2001/0040, London.

DoH (2001b) *A new bond of trust between patients and the NHS*. Alan Milburn speech to patient groups at the Kings Fund, Monday 29 January 2001. DOH Press Release 2001/0057, Department of Health, London.

Foster, C. (1998) Bolam: consolidation and clarification. *Health Care Risk Report*, 4 (5) April, 5–7.

Mason, J. K. & McCall Smith, R. A. (1999) *Law and Medical Ethics*, 5th Edn. Butterworths, London.

NAO (2000) National Audit Office Press Notice 24/00, NHS (England) Summarised Accounts 1998–99, at: http://www.nao.gov.uk/pn/9900356.htm. Assessed 28–02–01, also as referenced at HC 356, 1999/2000, 5 April 2000, The Stationery Office, London.

Stauch, M. & Wheat, K. with Tingle, J. H. (1998) *Sourcebook on Medical Law*. Cavendish Publishing, London.

The Times (2001) On-line Wednesday 17 January 2001, Lord Woolf's speech in full, assessed 18-01-01, http://www.thetimes.co.uk/article/0.2-69685.00.html.

Tingle, J. H. & Rodgers M. E. (1999) Clinical Guidelines, NICE and The Court of Appeal, *Nottingham Law School Journal*; 8 (2).

Tingle, J. H. (2000) The new, ambitious NHS Plan. *Health Care Risk Report*, 6 (10) October, 23–24.

Further reading

Eccles, M. & Grimshaw, J. (eds) (2000) *Clinical Guidelines From Conception to Use*. Radcliffe Medical Press, Oxford.
Furrow, B.R. (1999) Broadcasting clinical guidelines on the internet: will physicians tune in? *American Journal of Law and Medicine*, 25 (2 and 3), 403–21.
Jones, Michael A. (2000) *Textbook on Torts*, 7th edn. Blackstone Press, London.
Kennedy, Ian & Grubb, Andrew (2000) *Medical Law*. Butterworths, London.
Lugon, M. & Walker-Secker, Jonathan (eds) (1999) *Clinical Governance: Making it Happen*. The Royal Society of Medicine Press, London.
McHale, J, Tingle, J. & Peysner, J. (1998) *Law and Nursing*. Butterworth Heinemann, Oxford.
Wilson, J. & Tingle, J. (eds) (1999) *Clinical Risk Modification: A Route to Clinical Governance?* Butterworth Heinemann, Oxford.

Chapter 7

Conclusion: The Future of Clinical Governance for Healthcare Professionals

Rob McSherry and Paddy Pearce

In this book we have described why clinical governance was needed and what it is, together with its key components and how they relate to practicing clinicians, teams and organisations. The challenge for some healthcare organisations, teams and individuals is in resolving the many barriers affecting the successful implementation of clinical governance and in keeping up with the law as outlined in Chapter 6.

Given the importance with which the current government and no doubt future governments regard clinical governance, it goes without saying that it is here to stay. This is a concept or set of systems and processes that will be developed over time as it becomes engrained into the daily clinical and non-clinical practices of the NHS.

The desire of the healthcare professionals and public alike for the continuous improvement in clinical quality, in striving for excellence, further reinforces the need for clinical governance. Over the past 50 years we have witnessed many changes in the NHS, where some seem to have introduced a term 'changing things for the sake of change'. The changes attributed to clinical governance are somewhat different and cannot be viewed by the cynics as alluded to by Baker (2000) – the change for changing sake approach to health care policy – because clinical govern-ance is a broad framework that has encompassed many different strands of quality under a collective umbrella and made leaders of healthcare organisations responsible and accountable for assuring clinical and non-clinical quality.

Clinical governance provides NHS organisations, teams and individuals with a golden opportunity to make genuine and lasting improvements in the systems and process of care delivery as managerial and clinical responsibilities are harmonised.

The real opportunities and challenges facing some healthcare organisations, teams and individuals are in the development of realistic and achievable strategies that support their quest for the continuous quality improvement in providing excellent clinical care. Organisations, teams and individuals that are truly committed to clinical governance will realise that clinical governance is everybody's business, by ensuring a multidisciplinary and multiagency approach to the development of future services. For clinical governance to realise its potential the concept should be written into all job descriptions and contracts of employment for all NHS employees, an approach that reinforces the concept of ensuring accountability by all NHS staff for the provision of high quality care. Clinical governance must be included in the induction of all employees in ensuring a move towards the development, implementation and evaluation of the care, treatment or interventions they provide. A culture of openness, honesty and transparency with a willingness to learn from mistakes and share good practices needs to become the norm. The creation of such a culture will require time, commitment, vision, ambition and patience over a long period, where good communications, collaborations and partnerships between and within the systems and processes akin to clinical governance, along with the professions, are fundamental (Donaldson 2000).

The challenge for the future of healthcare organisations, teams and individuals is in resolving the barriers to clinical governance, barriers that are related to the founding principles of the NHS in ensuring universal access to a comprehensive service based on clinical need where equity of the services will be assured for all. These principles can only be assured in an organisation that is open to criticism and learns from its mistakes, as the recent media attention has taught the NHS. To ensure this open culture where expressing one's concerns or celebrating success becomes the norm, management and leadership that is democratic in nature requires development, where staff are valued and developed through the instigation of mutual partnerships and shared decision-making and ownership that reinforces the concept of accountability via the clinical governance framework. The task for individual healthcare professionals is in developing their knowledge, understanding and skills of applying the concept of clinical governance to their daily practice. Aligning clinical governance alongside their personal and professional development plans can only serve the professional well in the future. However, this will only become effective in an organisation that proactively seeks and values the true potential that clinical governance can unlock for their own organisation. Genuine sustained support and commitment needs to be guaranteed from the boards to the shop floor. The National Plan 2000 clearly states and stipulates the need for the adoption of a clinical governance framework by the organisation, team and individual by basing the entire document around assuring the continuous quality improvements of the NHS – a quality service that will be measured and evaluated against set national standards of care derived from the best available evidence published by NICE. The adherence to these standards along with the implementation of the clinical governance framework will be reviewed by CHi, which should be viewed as a supporting not a policing agency in evolving the future of the NHS.

As healthcare professionals concerned with providing the best standards of care to our patients and carers, we need to actively embrace this wonderful opportunity to partake in the modernisation of our NHS. Clinical governance is the vehicle to enable us to do this efficiently and effectively. So let us get involved with clinical governance in making a real and lasting difference for our NHS and patients in our care.

Good luck!

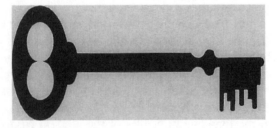

Clinical governance: The key to continuous quality improvements?

References

Baker, M. (2000) *Making Sense of the NHS White Papers*, 2nd edn. Radcliffe Medical Press Ltd, Oxford.

Donaldson, L. J. (2000) Clinical Governance; a mission to improve. *British Journal of Clinical Governance*, 5 (1), 6–8.

Useful websites

Commission for Health Improvements – www.chi.nhs.uk

National Institute for Clinical Excellence – www.nice.org.uk

University of Bradford Clinical Governance EBHC site (a site that has lots of links to many other useful sites) – www.brad.ac.uk/acad/health/pacg.htm

Clinical Governance: Quality in the New NHS original document – www.doh.gov.uk/pub/docs/doh/hsc065.pdf

Royal College of Nursing nursing site on clinical governance – www.rcn.org.uk/services/promote/quality.htm

The Wisdom Centre (a resource pack for clinical governance) – www.wisdomnet.co.uk/clingov.asp

Index

culture, organisational, 30–4, 37–8, 91,
92–7

definition of clinical governance,
16–21, 25, 115
demographic changes, 6
disadvantages of clinical governance,
23–4
doctors *see* medical profession

education *see* training
evaluation, evidence-based health care
and, 48
evidence-based health care, 45–8,
83–4
evolution of clinical governance, 13–15
expectations, raising of, 2, 4–5

force field theory, 99–100
functions style of management, 98
future of clinical governance, 126–8

government
   clinical governance and, 12, 16
   health policy changes, 1, 3–4
   quality of health care and, 2
Griffiths Report, 3

health care
   delivery systems
      changes in, 7
      non-clinical services and, 20–1
      performance management, 37–41,
      56, 72, 111
   evidence-based, 45–8, 83–4
   integrated, 73
   quality of *see* quality of health care
   technological changes, 6–7
health policy changes, 1, 3–4
human relationships management, 99

implementation of clinical governance,
60–78
   action plan, 67–8, 79–85
   barriers to, 89–113
   baseline assessment, 60, 61, 62–7

case studies, 68–76
healthcare organisations, 61–8
reasons for, 1–9
support for, 110–12
incident reporting, 40, 75
individual performance review (IPR),
40–1
information
   access to, 8, 9
   baseline assessment, 60, 61, 62–7
   quality, 49–54, 84
   see also clinical guidelines
integrated health care, 73
internal audit, 15, 73, 111
Investors in People award, 44

key components of clinical governance,
19–20, 29–34, 35, 56, 68
knowledge
   about clinical governance, 109–10
   about clinical guidelines, 121–3

leadership, 97, 101–3
league tables, 5
legal issues, 115–24
   clinical guidelines and, 120
      good practice, 123–4
      personal updating and, 121–3
   courts' determination of competent
      practice, 117–20
   definition of terms, 115
   litigation, 8–9, 116–17
life expectancy, 6
London Stock Exchange, 13

malpractice, 117–20, 121
management
   barriers to implementation of clinical
      governance, 97–101
   of change, 99–100
   changes in health care policy and,
      3–4
   clinical governance committees
      (CGCs), 61, 66, 67
   controls assurance and, 23
   functions style, 98